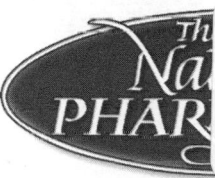

Inside—Find the Answers to These Questions and More

☑ Is it true that echinacea can reduce my cold symptoms and help me recover faster? (See page 52.)

☑ Is the herb St. John's wort effective for depression? (See page 176.)

☑ Can garlic really help lower my cholesterol? (See page 74.)

☑ Will kava help relieve my anxiety? (See page 128.)

☑ Can saw palmetto actually shrink an enlarged prostate? (See page 166.)

☑ Can feverfew reduce the nausea and pain of chronic migraine headaches? (See page 70.)

☑ Is there a natural treatment I can take to reduce ulcer pain? (See page 136.)

☑ Can ginkgo improve mental function in people with Alzheimer's disease? (See page 88.)

☑ Will ginger reduce nausea from motion sickness? (See page 83.)

☑ Can black cohosh relieve hot flashes and other menopausal symptoms? (See page 15.)

THE NATURAL PHARMACIST Library

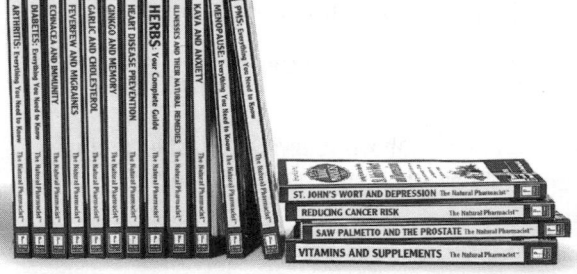

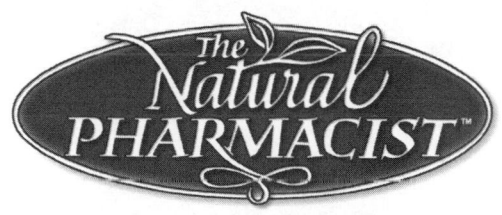

Your Complete Guide to Herbs

Steven Bratman, M.D.

Series Editors

Steven Bratman, M.D.
& David Kroll, Ph.D.

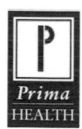

A DIVISION OF PRIMA PUBLISHING

Visit us online at www.thenaturalpharmacist.com

Library of Congress Cataloging-in-Publication Data

Bratman, Steven.
    Your complete guide to herbs / Steven Bratman.
      p.   cm. — (The natural pharmacist)
    Includes bibliographical references and index.
    ISBN 0-7615-1671-9
    1. Herbs—Therapeutic use. I. Title.
RM666.H33B726 1999
615.'321—dc21   98-22156
                                                                  CIP

00 01 02 HH 10 9 8 7 6 5 4 3 2
Printed in the United States of America

Visit us online at www.thenaturalpharmacist.com

Contents

Contents

What Makes This Book Different?

The interest in natural medicine has never been greater. According to the National Association of Chain Drug Stores, 65 million Americans are using natural supplements, and the number is growing! Yet, ironically, it is hard for the consumer to find trustworthy sources for balanced information about this emerging field. Why? Frankly, natural medicine has had a checkered history. From snake oil potions sold at the turn of the century to those books, magazines, and product catalogs that hype miracle cures today, this is a field where exaggerated claims have been the norm. Proponents of natural medicine have tended to abuse science, treating it more as a marketing tool than a means of discovering the truth.

But there is truth to be found. Studies of vitamins, minerals, and other food supplements have been with us since these nutritional substances were first discovered, and the level and quality of this science has grown dramatically in the last 20 years. Herbal medicine has been neglected in the United States, but in Europe, this, the oldest of all healing arts, has been the subject of tremendous and ongoing scientific interest.

At present, for a number of herbs and supplements, it is possible to give reasonably scientific answers to the questions: "How well does this work? How safe is it? What types of conditions is it best used for?"

THE NATURAL PHARMACIST series is designed to cut through the hype and tell you what we know and what we don't know about popular natural treatments. These books are more conservative than any others available, more honest about the weaknesses of natural approaches, more fair in their comparisons of natural and conventional treatments. You won't find any miracle cures here; but you will discover useful options that can help you become healthier.

Why Choose Natural Treatments?

Although the science behind natural medicine continues to grow, this is still a much less scientifically validated field than conventional medicine. You might ask, "Why should I resort to an herb that is only partly proven, when I could take a drug with solid science behind it?" There are at least three good reasons to consider natural alternatives.

First, some herbs and supplements offer benefits that are not matched by any conventional drug. Vitamin E is a good example. It appears to help prevent prostate cancer, a benefit that no standard medication can claim. Also, vitamin E almost certainly helps prevent heart disease. While there are standard drugs that also prevent heart disease, vitamin E works differently and may be able to complement many of the other approaches.

Another example is the herb milk thistle. Studies strongly suggest that this herb can protect the liver from injury. There is no pill or tablet your doctor can prescribe to do the same.

Even if the science behind some of these treatments is less than perfect, when the risks are low and the possible benefit high, a treatment may be worth trying. It is a little known fact that for many conventional treatments the science is less than perfect as well, and physicians must balance uncertain benefits against incompletely understood risks.

A second reason to consider natural therapies is that some may offer comparable benefits to drugs with fewer side effects. The herb St. John's wort is a good example. Reasonably strong scientific evidence suggests that this herb is an effective treatment for mild to moderate depression, while producing fewer side effects on average than conventional medications. Saw palmetto for benign enlargement of the prostate, ginkgo for relieving symptoms and perhaps slowing the progression of Alzheimer's disease, and glucosamine for osteoarthritis are other examples. This is not to say that herbs and supplements are completely harmless—they're not—but for most the level of risk is quite low.

Finally, there is a philosophical point to consider. For many people, it "feels" better to use a treatment that comes from nature instead of from a laboratory. Just as you might rather wear all-cotton clothing than polyester, or look at a mountain landscape rather than the skyscrapers of a downtown city, natural treatments may simply feel more compatible with your view of life. We can quibble endlessly about just what "natural" means and whether a certain treatment is "actually" natural or not, but such arguments are beside the point. The difference is in the feeling, and feelings matter. In fact, having a good feeling about taking an herb may lead you to use it more consistently than you would a prescription drug

Of course, at times synthetic drugs may be necessary and even lifesaving. But on many other occasions it may be quite reasonable to turn to an herb or supplement instead of a drug.

To make good decisions you need good information. Unfortunately, while hundreds of books on alternative medicine are published every year, many are highly misleading. The phrase "studies prove" is often used when the studies in question are so small or so badly conducted that they prove nothing at all. You may even find that the "data" from other books comes from studies with petri dishes and not real people!

You can't even assume that books written by well-known authors are scientifically sound. Many of these authors rely on secondary writers, leading to a game of "telephone" where misconceptions are passed around from book to book. And there's a strong tendency to exaggerate the power of natural remedies, whitewashing them with selective reporting.

THE NATURAL PHARMACIST series gives you the balanced information you need to make informed decisions about your health needs. Setting a new, high standard of accuracy and objectivity, these books take a realistic look at the herbs and supplements you read about in the news. You will encounter both favorable and unfavorable studies in these pages and will learn about both the benefits and the risks of natural treatments.

THE NATURAL PHARMACIST series is the source you can trust.

Steven Bratman, M.D.
David Kroll, Ph.D.

Introduction

For millennia, herbs were the primary medical treatment used around the world. Every great culture has found it worthwhile to devote considerable attention to cataloging the available herbs, evaluating methods of harvesting, storage, and preparation, as well as proper dosage, risks, and healing powers. However, with the rise of modern medicine, these ancient and diverse treatments gradually fell into disrepute and were replaced by chemicals either extracted from herbs or synthesized from other raw materials.

In the United States, herbs continued to be used by some mainstream physicians until World War II, but thereafter virtually no respected health-care professional took herbs seriously. They were regarded as superstitious relics from the dark ages of medicine; synthetic drugs and high-tech treatments seemed infinitely superior.

Herbal medicine became the sole province of the back-to-nature movement and the various health-care professions allied to it, such as naturopathy. In the 1980s, herbal medicine seemed close to losing its foothold even in the alternative world, swamped by a wave of interest in vitamins and food supplements.

The situation was much different in Europe. Mainstream medical practice never excluded the tradition of herbal treatment and major pharmaceutical houses continued to study herbs, eventually developing standardized extracts that could be easily tested in double-blind studies and sold for a significant profit. Herbs are widely prescribed by European physicians and form a major portion of the entire spectrum of drugs used in treatment.

In the last two years, this living European herbal tradition has suddenly made a dramatic impact in the United States. Not only popular magazines but even major medical journals have started to feature herbs such as St. John's wort, ginkgo, kava, and saw palmetto. The FDA has begun to look favorably on new drug applications for herbal medications, and the National Institutes of Health has funded a major study of St. John's wort.

However, amid all this excitement, perhaps the most important question may be forgotten: Why *do* herbs matter?

Why Do Herbs Matter?

Are herbs exciting just because they seem new and different? Are they a fashion, like Eurostyle kitchens or Swatch watches? Perhaps, but there are at least four good reasons to take a serious interest in herbal medicine: (1) We need to have access to any treatment that might work, (2) herbs are natural, (3) herbs are safer than drugs, and (4) herbs are gentler than drugs.

We Need to Have Access to Any Treatment That Might Work

When medicine began to create chemically purified drugs, one of its major sources was the herbs that had already been used for millennia. Quinine from cinchona bark, aspirin from salicin in white willow bark (and meadowsweet), digitalis from foxglove, and morphine from opium poppy are only a few of the many treatments given to us by the plant world. Even today, scientists are actively studying herbs with healing reputations in hopes of extracting the active principle, which will become a drug.

This method works fine when you can find an active ingredient. But in many herbs it seems that no individual purified constituent is effective. Apparently, the medicinal benefit depends on the influence of several separate ingredients. It isn't easy to turn such herbs into drugs.

Medical science has traditionally neglected herbs of this type for some very good reasons. These are described in detail under Standardization following. Briefly, if you can't find an active ingredient it's hard to know whether one batch of herb is as powerful as another. This is unacceptable to doctors, who demand reproducibility from their treatments.

Nonetheless, many very good herbal treatments simply can't be turned into drugs. If you are sick, you may not care too much about which ingredients of an herb are most effective, so long as the whole herb works. From your point of view, every potentially useful treatment may be worth considering, whether doctors are comfortable with it or not.

Some herbs without an obvious active ingredient appear to be as potent as drugs while producing fewer side effects. Saw palmetto for prostate enlargement and ginkgo for Alzheimer's disease are two major examples. If the drugs used for the same purpose produce too many side effects, you may be happier choosing an herb instead.

Not only can some herbs serve the same purpose as drugs, several of them provide unique benefits that are unmatched by any drug. The herb milk thistle, for example, can protect the liver from a wide range of toxins. No drug can boast the same effect. The same may be said for horse chestnut and its ability to reduce the pain and swelling of varicose veins, as well as echinacea and its ability to help you not only get over a cold significantly faster but sneeze less in the meantime. These benefits belong uniquely to herbs and not to any standard drug.

Taking care of one's health is sufficiently difficult that the more options one has to choose from the better. From this point of view, the arrival of European herbal treatments is simply an influx of choices neglected in the United States. However, this isn't the only reason to take an interest in herbal therapies.

Herbs Are Natural

While many people turn to herbs to increase their range of healing choices, others find herbs automatically preferable just because they are "natural": They would much rather take a natural product than a synthetic drug.

Most doctors don't have a lot of patience for this preference. They tend to get grumpy and say things like, "Just because it's natural doesn't mean it's good for you."

One major concern of physicians is that patients may falsely assume that *everything* natural is safe. Another influence is more subtle and psychological: Conventional medicine trains physicians to look on nature more as an enemy than a friend. Nature is always causing problems and doctors are supposed to try and fix those problems.

This pervasive attitude has led the medical profession to make some very strange recommendations. For example, from the 1920s until about the 1960s, medical authorities typically advised mothers to feed their babies artificial formula rather than breast milk. There was no scientific evidence for this advice. Formula just "felt" more scientific to doctors, while nursing a child seemed dangerously natural.

But to many nonphysicians, getting back in touch with nature is an important goal. Emotionally, herbs "feel" more wholesome than drugs. Even though there's no proof, for example, that St. John's wort is safer than Prozac, many people feel much more content to take the herb than the drug. It's a philosophical issue more than a rational one. Taking an herb feels like eating a food, while popping a chemical drug feels a bit self-polluting, despite the fact that both contain chemicals. Even when an herb causes a side effect, it doesn't feel as bad as a drug side effect. It's not logical, and it's hard to explain to someone who doesn't understand this perspective. But to those who do, it's self-evident.

Nonetheless, doctors are right to this extent: Just because an herb is natural doesn't mean that it's safe or effective. In the pages of this book, I will try to distinguish between romance and reality, and provide you with the latest scientific information for each herb discussed.

Herbs Are Safer Than Drugs

This is a controversial statement, but it has a considerable amount of truth behind it. To quickly see why, imagine the following experiment: Two people are blindfolded. One is taken behind the counter of a pharmacy to stand in front of a shelf of drugs. The other is placed before a rack of herbs. Then each grabs a bottle at random, removes the blindfold, and takes 20 times the suggested daily dose of whatever the bottle contains. Which person would you want to be?

It isn't difficult to decide. The person reaching for a drug would stand a really good chance of dying, while the one pulling an herb off the shelf would be very unlikely to suffer anything more than a wicked stomachache. The number of poisonings from medicinal herbs is overwhelmingly lower than those due to pharmaceutical medications, even in countries such as Germany, where herbs are very widely used.

In fairness, I should point out that German herbal preparations are made largely by pharmaceutical companies under much tighter standards than those of the United States. This avoids the problem of herbal contamination, when dangerous substances are packaged with or instead of the labeled herb, as has occurred more than once in the United States. (Such contamination is rare, however.) Also, since many drugs are used for critically ill patients, they tend to appear more dangerous statistically because the people who are taking them are so fragile to begin with. Finally, we know very little about potential herb/drug interactions.

Nonetheless, common medicinal herbs taken individually are definitely safer on average than drugs. Of course, some herbs are quite dangerous. Foxglove can kill you easily. But traditional herbalists long ago identified which herbs could cause serious immediate harm and concentrated on much safer plants. Most of the widely used medicinal herbs are quite benign, at least in the short run.

It should be kept in mind, however, that traditional usage can identify only common or immediate risks. It is much more difficult to identify risks that occur rarely, or only after a long period of use. Suppose that 1 in 10,000 ginkgo users develop bleeding problems.

A traditional herbalist would probably never treat anywhere near 10,000 people in a lifetime of practice, and thus would have no way of recognizing such a problem. A certain percentage of people are going to develop bleeding problems anyway. Only careful statistical records can tell us whether ginkgo causes an increased percentage of such problems, and traditional herbalists never kept such records.

On the other hand, we do keep track of the adverse-reaction statistics for drugs, and when rarely occurring adverse reactions are discovered it, makes the front pages of newspapers, *20/20,* and magazine covers. It is certainly possible that herbs cause similar problems, and we just don't know it yet.

Nonetheless, there is a strong faith among herbalists that herbs are safer than drugs. The origin of this belief is more emotional and spiritual than purely rational—an intuitive sense that God created herbs to heal both men and beasts. Nature doctors of the nineteenth century explicitly declared that medicine made by God is always superior to medicine made by man, and they hurled this charge against chemical drugs, purified herbal extracts, and, ironically, even vitamins.

Modern proponents of herbal medicine seldom use this argument directly. However, if you listen closely you'll discover that it underlies their more reasoned explanations. Belief in the superiority of herbs is really a form of faith.

But it's not difficult to think of a perfectly reasonable scientific explanation for the apparent safety of herbs, one that does not require faith. It goes as follows: Even though plants don't have any evolutionary compulsion to cure animals, there *would* be an evolutionary advantage to animals that could cure themselves of illnesses by eating appropriate plants.

Animals evolved in a sea of plants, and developed their biochemical makeup in relation to what was available as food. Perhaps part of this evolution also included a responsiveness to various plant chemicals for healing purposes. Just as animals instinctively appreciate salt licks and natural mineral deposits when they are short on necessary nutrients, there may be a built-in mechanism that helps them (and presumably humans as well) find the herbs to take when sick. Our bodies would therefore evolve to make use of the flavonoids, diterpenes, steroids, and alkaloids so commonly found in medicinal plants. And we would evolve defenses against the most common plant poisons. This is pure speculation, of course, but it does make sense. Without invoking any spiritual beliefs, it gives meaning to the notion that herbs are somehow "better for you than drugs." We did not evolve in a sea of drugs.

Nonetheless, some herbs have proven to be dangerous. The more extensive the safety studies performed on an herb, the safer I feel about recommending it. Many of the most popular herbs have been evaluated fairly thoroughly from a safety point of view. Other herbs have not been so evaluated, but based on extensive use as food, the FDA has placed them on its GRAS (generally regarded as safe) list. Unfortunately, the GRAS list can be misleading. It simply assures the safety of some herbs at concentrations used primarily as food flavorings, and these "doses" are often well below those used for medicinal purposes. So you can't take it as a complete reassurance.

The bottom line is that safety with medicinal herbs is not guaranteed, although on average they are probably relatively safe.

Herbs Are Gentler Than Drugs

Herbs are widely described as gentle treatments, because they tend to cause few side effects. Of course, this is not true of all herbs. If you read literature from the nineteenth century, you'll find recommendations for herbal treatments with very severe side effects indeed. For example, the herb lobelia was commonly recommended to be taken to the point of severe vomiting. But most medicinal herbs used today produce practically no side effects at all. The most common problems that do occur are nonspecific symptoms, such as occasional allergic reactions as well as mild digestive distress.

To be fair, some of the newest drugs on the market are remarkably side-effect free as well. But, on average, the medicinal herbs described in this book produce fewer unpleasant reactions than standard medications.

How Well Do Herbs Really Work?

Just because herbs are generally safe and relatively side-effect free doesn't mean they are effective. In fact, it wouldn't be unreasonable to expect herbs to be less effective on average than drugs precisely because they are milder, and in many cases this is true. Some herbs, however, are just as powerful as conventional medications.

The only reliable proof that an herb is effective is a type of study called a *double-blind placebo-controlled trial.* In this kind of research, half the participants are given real treatment and the other half take a placebo. What makes the studies "blind" is that neither doctor nor patient knows which is which. If properly designed, this type of study thoroughly eliminates the power of suggestion and gives solid information on the effectiveness of a treatment.

Studies that aren't blinded are called *open studies,* and you have to take their results with a grain of salt. The influence of suggestion is remarkably powerful. Phony pills frequently produce dramatic and long-lasting results in more than 50% of the people who take them and also cause side effects ranging from headaches to nausea! If you want to know what a treatment is doing apart from the effects of suggestion, you really need double-blind studies.

Also, such studies have to be reasonably large to prove much. Treatments that produce a relatively mild effect at best, such as saw palmetto for prostate enlargement, need to include at least 100 people to make a good case, and 300 participants would be a lot better. Dramatically effective treatments can prove themselves in somewhat smaller trials. However, research involving 20 or fewer people generally doesn't prove anything at all. If you flip a coin 20 times, chances are pretty good that the number of heads and tails won't come out even, "proving" that the coin is biased. One of my daughter's friends performed the experiment and counted 12 heads and 8 tails. To her, this proved that heads were more likely with that penny by a full 50%! Too many studies reported in the media are about as conclusive as this one.

Many other kinds of studies also don't prove much. One example is the famous *in vitro,* or test-tube, study. Magazines never seem to tire of reporting old studies that found garlic capable of killing bacteria in test tubes. The obvious but incorrect conclusion is that when you eat garlic, it acts as an antiobiotic. However, if you pour vine-gar, orange juice, or bleach in a test tube, any of them will also kill bacteria. But these liquids don't work the same way when you drink them! Test-tube studies do not account for the fact that an herb taken orally must be absorbed into the bloodstream, survive processing by the liver, and still manage to be effective when diluted by the fluids of the body. It's a long leap from a test tube to a real treatment. In vitro studies are really only spurs to further research: They don't prove that a treatment is effective in real life.

There are many other examples of potentially misleading research. Studies that use injections instead of oral dosing can't be fully trusted because an injected substance doesn't have to run the gauntlet of the digestive tract. Studies that focus on components of herbs rather than the herbs themselves can't be relied on because concentrated preparations of individual herb constituents frequently produce effects, both good and bad, that do not occur with the whole herb. Furthermore, there are many basic scientific investigations that show *how* an herb might work but not that it *does* work. For example, echinacea has been shown to activate white blood cells, but this does not guarantee that it strengthens the immune system. Sugar-cane activates white blood cells too. Although they provide a great deal of useful information, animal studies, too, are potentially misleading because animal physiology can be very different from human physiology.

Fortunately, for many herbs, there is a reasonable body of double-blind research (almost all of it from Europe). Based on this information, we can say with some certainty that saw palmetto is as good as or better than standard drugs for the treatment of benign prostate enlargement. And there is very little doubt that St. John's wort (at least in the tested formulation) is effective for about 60% of people with mild to moderate depression.

Perhaps eight of the herbs described in this book have strong evidence behind them, and two dozen more have some double-blind evidence. As for the rest, keep in mind that just because an herb hasn't been proven to work doesn't mean that it doesn't work. We simply don't know yet.

Generally, the most scientifically documented herbal treatments are the popular European herbal extracts. However, there are literally thousands of other medicinal herbs in wide use, and exciting new herbal options are constantly arriving from India, China, the former Soviet Union, the Amazon basin, and many other exotic locales. In comparison with the modern European herbs, the scientific evidence for these other treatments is rather weak. There are seldom good double-blind studies available, and the safety of these herbs is generally not well documented. Nonetheless, many of these treatments have the weight of long tradition behind them and, in many cases, some promising preliminary evidence. These herbs are worth watching closely, because many are under intensive study at the present time and may become the scientifically verified herbal medications of the next decade. Throughout this book I will report whatever information is available about the effectiveness of herbs, whether from science, tradition, or practical experience.

One final point: It's common to romanticize herbal medicine and exaggerate its powers. After writing a book on St. John's wort, I was prompted by a radio interviewer to tell the audience "how St. John's wort gets to the root of depression and heals it from within." Unfortunately, I couldn't oblige him. St. John's wort is a very good antidepressant with a terrific side-effects profile, but it doesn't "heal" depression. Psychotherapy may be able to heal depression sometimes, but St. John's wort, like Prozac, only alleviates symptoms. This is a great contribution in itself. It doesn't need to be puffed up into something miraculous.

Herbs can be very useful but they are seldom miracle cures. The only real miracle is life itself; medical treatments, whether conventional or alternative, simply consist of the best we can do to confront the complex problems of health and illness.

How Are Herbs Sold?

In the United States, herbs are sold as food supplements only (except for a few approved herbal drugs, such as cascara for constipation). Manufacturers are not allowed to label herbs with a description telling what diseases they may treat. For example, bottles of St. John's wort pills cannot state "to be used for mild to moderate depression." Such a statement would make the herb into a drug, and drugs have to go through a complex and expensive approval process. Instead, products can list only vague claims, such as "supports the function of the nervous system."

However, in Europe, the status of herbs corresponds more closely to that of over-the-counter (OTC) drugs. Germany has the most organized system of any European country. In 1978, the German Federal Health Agency organized a special commission to evaluate the safety and efficacy of medicinal herbs. The Commission E Monographs were the outcome of this effort, consisting of 300 articles on the most medically important herbal preparations. These monographs serve as the basis for the medical usage of herbs within the German health-care system, allowing them to be prescribed by physicians. Whenever they are available, the recommendations of Commission E will be cited in the discussion of individual herbs.

Since the original Commission E Monographs were drafted, the level of scientific investigation into herbal medications has continued to grow. Furthermore, some herbs are neglected in Germany, but well studied in France, Italy, or the United Kingdom. Gathered together, all this information gives modern European herbal medicine a substantial scientific foundation.

Interestingly, in the 1960s, a commission similar to Commission E was established in the United States to evaluate OTC medications that had been marketed prior to the 1962 enactment of our modern drug-testing process. The U.S. National Academy of Sciences Commission reviewed the safety and efficacy data for OTC medicines, allowing only those with convincing data to continue to be sold as "drugs." A majority of today's OTC medicines were approved by this type of review, rather than strict double-blind testing. Some herbs are included, such as *Cascara sagrada* for constipation.

Presently, a few herb manufacturers have presented their special herb formulations to the FDA to start the process of approval. In a few years, we will no doubt see some of the best-documented herbs appear as approved drugs. In the meantime, they are food supplements, widely available but with little oversight and almost incomprensible labeling.

How Should I Take Herbs?

Herbs present one annoying problem that simply does not exist with drugs. When manufacturers produce aspirin tablets, they can easily list the milligrams of aspirin present in each pill. Aspirin is a single chemical, acetyl-salicylic acid. Provided the manufacturer is honest, one pill labeled "325 mg aspirin" is remarkably like another.

But herbs are not single chemicals. They were recently living plants, composed of thousands of different chemicals, whose exact proportion varies widely from crop to crop. Numerous factors affect the constituents of herbs, including growing conditions (such as weather, sunlight, quality of the soil, time of harvest), duration and method of storage, and technique of preparation (whether air-drying, freeze-drying, or chemical extraction). Because of the great potential for variation, there's no good way to pronounce one tablet equivalent to another. If we knew the active ingredient, we could simply measure its level. But, in the great majority of cases, the active ingredient of medicinal herbs is unknown. This leaves even the most well-intentioned of manufacturers helpless to guarantee the potency of their products.

In the old days, herbalists simply harvested their herbs according to the lore they had been taught, basing their judgment of potency by taste, smell, and past experience. Some herb companies do so even today. The only problem with this method is that it isn't terribly verifiable. How can you know when you buy an herb "carefully selected by our master herbalists" that (1) those master herbalists know what to look for and (2) those master herbalists really exist and aren't just a figment of Madison Avenue.

Standardization

Many of the major European herb manufacturers are pharmaceutical companies. In the habit of producing scientifically reproducible products, these companies could not rest content hiring people to smell and taste the herbs. They felt compelled to develop a more scientifically reliable process. This desire led to the development of what are called *standardized herbal extracts*, a form of herbal preparation that stands halfway between a whole herb and a drug. Such preparations are not as completely reproducible as aspirin, but much more so than raw willow bark, and they've become increasingly popular in the United States as well.

A standardized herbal extract is made according to a defined process. For example, the manufacturers may harvest St. John's wort in July, grind up the whole plant, soak the ground herb for exactly 11 hours in a hot mixture of 30% alcohol and water, and then strain off the plant product. Next, they "boil down" the extracted liquid until it contains a certain percentage of some ingredient.

This does not have to be the active ingredient. In fact, it usually isn't. It's just a tag, or a handle. Hopefully, if it is present in a fixed concentration, other unknown but important ingredients will also be present in a roughly fixed percentage. For St. John's wort, "hypericin" is the usual tag ingredient, standardized to a concentration of 0.3%. (Contrary to some news reports, hypericin is not the active ingredient in St. John's wort. By itself, hypericin is not believed to be an effective antidepressant at all. Another constituent named hyperforin is showing promise, however.)

Standardized extracts can then be used in scientific studies with some expectation that each batch will be as strong as the other. For example, several studies have found that a particular standardized extract of ginkgo can improve symptoms of Alzheimer's disease. It seems quite likely that any sample of this certain extract, whether purchased in Germany or the United States, will prove just as effective a treatment.

It's important to keep in mind that when such a study demonstrates the therapeutic effect of a certain herbal extract, the results don't necessarily apply to any other formulation of the same herb. The method of extraction used to standardize the herb concentrates certain substances and not others, and since the active ingredients are unknown, different types of herbal preparations may not be equivalent. If another process uses a higher percentage of alcohol, or substitutes methanol for ethanol, for example, or boils the extract at a higher or lower temperature, the final product may either be more or less effective than the one studied.

Unfortunately, often manufacturers of herbs, such as ginkgo, use the results of studies performed on different formulations than the one they sell. "Ginkgo is proven to help Alzheimer's," they say, and then market a product manufactured completely differently. This is called "borrowing science," and there is no guarantee that it leads to correct claims.

If a drug company wants to manufacture a generic version of a drug that has lost its patent, it will also borrow the science from the original patented drug. But it's not terribly difficult to assure equivalence between generic and name brand drugs because the active ingredients are known, and there is usually only one ingredient per tablet. With the thousands of compounds present in herbs, coupled with the lack of knowledge regarding which is most important, assuring equivalence is essentially impossible. We really only know the effectiveness of the precise herb formulation used in the study.

Many of the actual European herbal products used in studies are now available in the United States. Furthermore, U.S. manufacturers are starting to imitate European extraction methods and offer essentially similar products. Herbs such as these may be your best bet.

But remember that there is no reason to believe unstandardized products won't work. We just usually lack scientific evidence to show that they do work, and there may be huge differences from batch to batch. Standardization increases reproducibility but not necessarily effectiveness.

For example, in a pair of recent studies of using the herb feverfew to treat migraine headaches, whole leaf turned out to be more effective than a standardized extract. (See the discussion under Feverfew in the text.) And an expert at one major herb company told me confidentially that although they have begun to produce standardized forms of St. John's wort to satisfy the public, their older unstandardized preparation actually works better!

The bottom line is this: If you take an herb and it doesn't seem to work, the problem may not be with the herb itself, but with the preparation. You may simply have to try more than one brand to find what works best for you.

Can I Take Herbs and Drugs at the Same Time?

Unfortunately, not very much is known about herb/drug interactions. Few adverse herb/drug reactions have ever been reported, but it's quite possible and even likely that there will be problems yet to be discovered.

For each herb discussed in this book, I describe all known or suspected drug interactions. Sometimes the suspected problems are highly theoretical, more a matter of extreme prudence than actual likelihood. You and your physician will have to decide how seriously to take these hypothetical concerns. Other concerns are based on documented reports. Even in these cases, it is hard to be sure whether the herb was really at fault, or whether it was a coincidence.

One way in which drugs and herbs (and any drug combination in general) may interact is through effects on the liver. Over the millions of years of human history, we have ingested numerous chemicals from natural sources that our bodies have had to learn to process. It is primarily the liver that handles these chemicals, neutralizing or helping to eliminate dangerous ones. Many medications are also processed by the liver. The proper dose of medication is in part determined by how fast your liver can remove it. The faster your liver breaks down a drug, the more you have to take.

Problems may arise when an herb (or another drug) interferes with the rate at which your liver processes a medication. The herb may contain a substance that keeps the liver so busy it doesn't attend to your medication. This can lead to drug levels rising in your blood, perhaps to potentially toxic levels. The opposite effect is also possible: An herb may "rev" up the liver so that it attacks a drug with increased effectiveness, reducing its level in your blood and perhaps rendering it ineffective.

While large databases exist for your doctor and pharmacist to assess drug/drug metabolic interactions, the amount of information on herb/drug interactions is comparatively poor. Therefore, when taking an herb with any drug, it is important to pay attention to either any increase in drug side effects or even the loss of a drug's beneficial effect. Most of the time, there will be no problems. But it is always in your best interest to let your doctor or pharmacist know of any new supplements that you are taking any time you have a problem with your prescribed medications. At the very least, this can contribute to our knowledge on this important subject.

One drug definitely presents a risk if combined with herbs: Coumadin, or warfarin. This powerful blood thinner is fairly dangerous, and even ordinary foods can interact with it. If you decide to take a new herb while on Coumadin, you absolutely must inform your doctor and take a blood-coagulation test.

Other drugs to worry about are the narrow therapeutic index (NTI) agents, such as digitalis. An NTI drug has a relatively narrow range, or window, between amounts that cause the desired effect and amounts that are toxic. There is at least one report of ginseng raising digitalis levels. Another example is the asthma drug theophylline. Although theophylline has fallen out of favor—it is an NTI drug and there are non-NTI alternatives available—its use is not unheard of. St. John's wort may interfere with its levels. When taking an NTI drug, don't use any herbal products (or OTC medications!) without first checking with your doctor or pharmacist.

Another potential problem arises if you take an herb and a drug that both produce the same desired effect. You may be trying to see if the herb can help reduce the dosage of drug you need. Alternatively, you may be trying to switch from a drug to an herb and wish to overlap treatments during a transition period. Many people do this with Prozac and St. John's wort, for example, cutting the Prozac to half strength for a couple of weeks while starting the herb.

However, no one knows if this approach is truly safe. There is at least a possibility that the combined result will be too much of a good thing. There are concerns that Prozac and St. John's wort combined together could elevate serotonin too much, causing problems known as serotonergic syndrome. For another example, you may wish to add *Coleus forskohlii* to drug treatment for your high blood pressure in order to achieve an improved effect. However, it's possible that your blood pressure will fall too low. You need to add the herbal treatment in a very low dose at first, and then gradually increase it while monitoring the effect. A doctor's supervision is essential.

Why Are Chinese Herb Combinations Discussed Separately?

At the end of this book, there is a small section on Chinese herb combinations. This is just the briefest of introductions into a very different approach to herbal medicine. Although several individual herbs used in these combinations are discussed in the main body of the text, Chinese herb combinations belong in a class of their own.

Traditional Chinese herbology is very different from the herbal medicine of most of the rest of the world. Instead of using herbs alone, it almost always combines them in complex and very individualized formulas. When properly performed, Chinese herbal medicine treats the person, rather than the disease, so it isn't really possible to say that formula A is for migraines and formula B is for bladder infections. Each formula belongs only and specifically to the person it's designed for.

It takes a great deal of training to learn how to use Chinese herbal medicine, far too much for most people to self-prescribe. You need to seek the services of a competent practitioner. However, a few Chinese formulas can be used without special training, and in the Chinese Patent Formulas section I introduce some of the most common ones. Keep in mind that there is very little science behind the use of these treatments, whether for safety or effectiveness.

When Should I Self-Treat with Herbs, and When Should I Seek Professional Advice?

In general, herbal medicine is most appropriate for conditions of a mild to moderate nature. If you do have a serious condition, such as diabetes or angina, herbs may still be useful, but they will most likely serve as an addition to drug therapy rather than a replacement for it. In such cases, it is always necessary to inform your physician that you want to take herbs. As mentioned earlier, sometimes herbs and drugs can add up together to create too strong an effect.

But if your physician describes your medical condition as relatively non-dangerous, or only dangerous if left untreated for many years, you can explore the world of herbal medicine with confidence. Perhaps you will find an effective and side-effect-free treatment that suits you perfectly. For now, let's enter the world of herbs.

ALOE

(ALOE VERA)

Principal Proposed Uses

Topical uses: Wound and burn healing

Oral uses: AIDS, diabetes, asthma, ulcers, immune weakness

The succulent aloe plant has been valued since prehistoric times for the treatment of burns, wound infections, and other skin problems. Medicinal aloe is pictured in an ancient cave painting in South Africa, and Alexander the Great is said to have captured an island off Somalia for the sole purpose of possessing the luxurious crop of aloe found there.

Most uses of aloe refer to the gel inside its cactus-like leaves. However, the skin of the leaves themselves can be condensed to form a sticky substance known as "drug aloe" or "aloes." It is a powerful laxative, and an unpleasant one. The uses described below refer only to aloe gel.

What Is Aloe Used for Today?

I suspect millions of people (including myself) would swear by their own experience that applying aloe to the skin can drastically reduce the time it takes for a burn to heal. Unfortunately there have never been any properly designed scientific studies that can tell us just how effective aloe really is.[1]

Topical aloe gel also appears to improve the rate of healing of minor cuts and scrapes. However, one report suggests that aloe can actually impair healing in severe wounds.[2]

Oral *Aloe vera* is also sometimes recommended to treat AIDS, diabetes, asthma, stomach ulcers, and general immune weakness. While the evidence for benefit in these conditions is slight to nonexistent, one of the constituents of aloe, acemannan, does seem to possess numerous interesting effects. Test-tube and animal studies suggest that it may stimulate immunity and inhibit the growth of viruses.[3,4,5] However, it remains to be discovered whether this preliminary research will translate into actual benefits in human beings. Aloe vera is definitely not a proven treatment for any of these conditions.

Dosage

For sunburn and other minor burns, smear aloe gel liberally on the affected area.

For internal use in treating AIDS and other conditions, some authorities recommend a dose of aloe standardized to provide 800 to 1,600 mg of the substance acemannan daily.

Safety Issues

Other than occasional allergic reactions, no serious problems have been reported with aloe gel, whether used internally or externally. However, comprehensive safety studies are lacking. Safety in young children, pregnant or nursing women, or those with severe liver or kidney disease is not established.

ANDROGRAPHIS

(ANDROGRAPHIS PANICULATA)

Principal Proposed Uses

Colds (shortening duration and reducing symptoms)

Andrographis is a shrub found throughout India and other Asian countries that is sometimes called "Indian echinacea."

It has been used historically in epidemics, including the Indian flu epidemic in 1919, during which andrographis was credited with stopping the spread of the disease.[1]

What Is Andrographis Used for Today?

Over the last decade, andrographis has become popular in Scandinavia as a treatment for colds. It is beginning to become available in the United States as well.

What Is the Scientific Evidence for Andrographis?

A few well-designed, double-blind studies that found andrographis to be effective have recently been published in English. The evidence suggests that andrographis reduces the severity of symptoms and shortens the length of colds.

One recent, double-blind clinical study of andrographis involved 50 people with colds who received either andrographis or placebo.[2] The results showed that 55% of the treated participants reported that their colds were less intense than usual, while only 19% of those in the placebo group stated this. About 75% of the treated individuals were well after 5 days, compared to less than 40% in the placebo group. These differences are statistically significant and provide meaningful evidence that andrographis is effective.

Another study of 59 people found similar results.[3] Participants received either 1,200 mg of andrographis (standardized to 4% *andrographolides*) or placebo, and were evaluated for the severity of cold symptoms such as fatigue, sore muscles, runny nose, headache, and lymph node swelling. By the fourth day of the study, the andrographis group showed significant improvement in most of the cold symptoms, including sore throat, muscle aches, and fatigue, as compared to the placebo group.

Finally, a double-blind study involving 152 adults compared the effectiveness of andrographis (in doses of 3 g per day or 6 g per day, for 7 days) to acetaminophen for the treatment of sore throat and fever. The higher dose of andrographis (6 g) decreased symptoms of fever and throat pain, as did acetaminophen, while the lower dose of andrographis (3 g) did not.

There were no significant side effects in either group.[4]

Dosage

A typical dosage of andrographis is 400 mg 3 times a day. Doses as high as 1,000 to 2,000 mg 3 times daily have been used in some studies. Andrographis is usually standardized to its content of andrographolide, typically 4 to 6%.

Safety Issues

Andrographis has not been associated with any side effects in human studies, although animal studies raise concerns about its effects on fertility. In the 59-person study mentioned earlier, participants were monitored for changes in liver function, blood counts, kidney function, and other laboratory measures of toxicity.[5] No problems were found.

However, some studies have raised concerns that andrographis may impair fertility. One study showed that male rats became infertile when fed 20 mg of andrographis powder daily.[6] In this case, the rats stopped producing sperm and showed physical changes in some of the testicular cells involved in sperm production. Researchers also detected evidence of degeneration of other anatomical structures in the testicles. However, another study showed no evidence of testicular toxicity in male rats that were given up to 1 g per kilogram body weight daily for 60 days, so this issue remains unclear.[7]

One group of female mice also did not fare well on high dosages of andrographis.[8] When fed 2 g per kilogram body weight daily for 6 weeks (thousands of times higher than the usual human dose), all female mice failed to get pregnant when mated with males of proven fertility. Meanwhile, of the control females, 95.2% got pregnant when mated with a similar group of male mice.

While andrographis is probably not a useful form of birth control, these results are worrisome and suggest the need for more research. Safety in young children, pregnant or nursing women, or those with severe liver or kidney disease is not established.

ASHWAGANDA

(WITHANIA SOMNIFERUM)

Principal Proposed Uses

Adaptogen (improve ability to withstand stress)

Other Proposed Uses

Improve exercise ability, immunity, sexual capacity, and fertility

Ashwaganda is sometimes called "Indian ginseng," not because it's related botanically (it's closer to potatoes and tomatoes), but because its uses are similar. Like ginseng, ashwaganda is a "tonic herb" traditionally believed capable of generally strengthening the body. However, it is believed to be milder and less stimulating than ginseng.

What Is Ashwaganda Used for Today?

Modern herbalists classify ashwaganda as an adaptogen, a substance that increases the body's ability to withstand stress of all types. (See Ginseng for more information on adaptogens.)

Like other adaptogens, ashwaganda is said to improve physical energy, strengthen immunity, and increase sexual capacity. It is also said to act as a fertility drug.

Highly preliminary studies suggest that ashwaganda may reduce the negative effects of stress, inhibit inflammation, lower cholesterol, increase sexual performance, produce mild sedation, increase hemoglobin levels, and inhibit tumor growth.[1-4] Further studies remain to be performed to evaluate these potential benefits.

Dosage

A typical dosage of ashwaganda is 1 teaspoon of powder twice a day, boiled in milk or water. Herbalists often recommend that those who are young or especially weak should take a lower dosage.

Safety Issues

Although formal scientific safety studies have not been completed, ashwaganda appears to be safe when taken in normal doses. However, because some of the constituents of ashwaganda can make you drowsy, it should not be combined with sedative drugs. The herb may also have some steroid-like activity at high dosages. Safety in young children, pregnant or nursing women, or those with severe liver or kidney disease is not established.

ASTRAGALUS

(ASTRAGALUS MEMBRANACEUS)

Principal Proposed Uses

Strengthen immunity (against cold, flus, and other illnesses)

Other Proposed Uses

Atherosclerosis, high blood pressure, hyperthyroidism, insomnia, diabetes, chronic active hepatitis, genital herpes, AIDS, chemotherapy side effects

Dried and sliced thin, the root of the astragalus plant is a common component of traditional Chinese herbal formulas. According to Chinese medical theory, astragalus "strengthens the spleen, blood and Qi, raises the yang Qi of the spleen and stomach, and stabilizes the exterior."[1] Don't worry if you didn't understand what you just read, because without many months of training in the unique Chinese approach to illness, there's no way you could have. Suffice it to say that the traditional understanding of the way astragalus works is different from the way it tends to be presented today.

What Is Astragalus Used for Today?

In the United States, astragalus has been presented as an immune stimulant useful for treating colds and flus. Many people have come to believe that they should take astragalus, like echinacea, at the first sign of a cold.

The belief that astragalus can strengthen the immunity has its basis in Chinese tradition. The expression "stabilize the exterior" means helping to create a "defensive shield" against infection.

However, according to Chinese healing tradition, astragalus formulas should not be taken during the early stage of infections. To do so is said to resemble "locking the chicken-coop with the fox inside," causing the infection to be "driven deeper."

Rather, astragalus is supposedly only appropriate for use while you're healthy, for the purpose of preventing future illnesses. Since it was the Chinese who first developed astragalus, perhaps these traditions should be taken seriously.

What Is the Scientific Evidence for Astragalus?

Although tradition suggests that astragalus should always be used in combination with other herbs, modern Chinese investigators have found various intriguing effects when astragalus is taken by itself. Extracts of astragalus have been shown to stimulate parts of the immune system in mice and humans, and to increase the survival time of mice infected with various diseases.[2,3] Preliminary research also suggests that astragalus might be useful in treating atherosclerosis, hyperthyroidism, high blood pressure, insomnia, diabetes, chronic active hepatitis, genital herpes, AIDS, and the side effects of cancer chemotherapy.[4–9] However, none of these suggestions can be regarded as proven.

Dosage

A typical daily dosage of astragalus involves boiling 9 to 30 g of dried root to make tea. Newer products use an alcohol-and-water extraction method to produce an extract standardized to astragaloside content, although there is no consensus on the proper percentage.

Safety Issues

Astragalus appears to be relatively nontoxic. High one-time doses, as well as long-term administration, have not caused significant harmful effects.[10] Side effects are rare and generally limited to the usual mild gastrointestinal distress or allergic reactions.

As mentioned above, traditional Chinese medicine warns against using astragalus in cases of acute infections. Other traditional contraindications include "deficient yin patterns with heat signs" and "exterior excess heat patterns." Because understanding what these mean would require an extensive education in Chinese medicine, I recommend using astragalus only under the supervision of a qualified Chinese herbalist.

Safety in young children, pregnant or nursing women, or those with severe liver or kidney disease is not established.

BILBERRY

(VACCINIUM MYRTILLUS)

Principal Proposed Uses

Eye problems (e.g., poor night vision, diabetic retinopathy, prevention of cataracts, prevention and treatment of macular degeneration)

Strengthen blood vessels (e.g., varicose veins, easy bruising, prevention of post-surgical bleeding)

Often called European blueberry, bilberry is closely related to American blueberry, cranberry, and huckleberry. Its meat is creamy white instead of purple, but it is traditionally used, like blueberries, in the preparation of jams, pies, cobblers, and cakes.

Bilberry fruit also has a long medicinal history. In the twelfth century, Abbess Hildegard of Bingen wrote of bilberry's usefulness for inducing menstruation. Over subsequent centuries, the list of uses for bilberry grew to include a bewildering variety of possible uses, from bladder stones to typhoid fever.

What Is Bilberry Used for Today?

The modern use of bilberry dates back to World War II, when British Royal Air Force pilots reported that a good dose of bilberry jam just prior to a mission improved their night vision, often dramatically. After the war, medical researchers investigated the constituents of bilberry and subsequently recommended it for a variety of eye disorders.

Bilberry is used throughout Europe today for the treatment of poor night vision and day blindness, for which it is believed to be significantly helpful. Regular use of bilberry is also thought to help prevent or treat other eye diseases such as macular degeneration, diabetic retinopathy, and cataracts.

Scientific research also found that bilberry contains biologically powerful substances known as anthocyanosides. Evidence suggests that anthocyanosides strengthen the walls of blood vessels, reduce inflammation and generally stabilize all tissues containing collagen (such as tendons, ligaments, and cartilage).[1–5] Grape seed contains related substances with similar properties. However, bilberry's anthocyanosides have a special attraction to the retina, which may explain this herb's apparent usefulness in eye diseases.[6]

There is also some evidence that bilberry can be useful for varicose veins. European physicians additionally believe that bilberry's blood vessel stabilizing properties also make it useful as a treatment before surgery to reduce bleeding complications, as well as for other blood-vessel problems such as easy bruising, but the evidence as yet is only suggestive.

What Is the Scientific Evidence for Bilberry?

Although bilberry is widely used by physicians in Europe based on research performed in the 1960s and earlier, all together the research into bilberry is not yet up to modern standards. However, this is an active area of research, and you can expect new information to be available soon.

Night Vision

Two early controlled, but not double-blind, studies of bilberry found that the herb improved night vision.[7] A more recent double-blind placebo-controlled study on 40 healthy subjects found that a single dose of bilberry extract improved visual response for 2 hours.[8]

Visual benefits have also been reported in numerous, more recent trials, but these studies did not use a placebo control group.[9,10,11]

Diabetic Retinopathy

A double-blind placebo-controlled trial of bilberry extract in 14 people with damage to the retina caused by diabetes and/or hypertension found significant improvements observable by ophthalmoscopic examination (looking in the eye with a machine) and angiography (examining the blood vessels).[12] However, this was a very preliminary study.

Other studies have found similar results, but they were not double-blind.[13,14] (For more information on diabetes, see *The Natural Pharmacist Guide to Diabetes*.)

Cataracts

Although antioxidants in general are believed to help prevent cataracts, direct research into bilberry's effects appears to be limited to one human study that combined the herb with vitamin E.[15] The combination was effective, but whether it was the herb or the vitamin that helped most remains unclear.

Varicose Veins

In a placebo-controlled study that followed 60 people with varicose veins (technically, venous insufficiency) for 30 days, bilberry extract resulted in a significant decrease in pain and swelling.[16] Similar results were seen in a 30-day double-blind trial involving 47 individuals.[17] Numerous other studies have yielded similarly positive results, although they did not use a placebo group.[18,19] However, there is better evidence for horse chestnut, grape seed, and gotu kola (see those sections for more information).

Dosage

The standard dosage of bilberry is 120 to 240 mg twice daily of an extract standardized to contain 25% anthocyanosides.

Safety Issues

Bilberry is a food and as such is quite safe. Enormous quantities have been administered to rats without toxic effects.[20,21] One study of 2,295 people given bilberry extract found a 4% incidence of side effects such as mild digestive distress, skin rashes, and drowsiness.[22] Although safety in pregnancy has not been proven, studies have enrolled pregnant women.[23] Safety in young children, nursing women, or those with severe liver or kidney disease is not known. There are no known drug interactions.

BITTER MELON
(MOMORDICA CHARANTIA)

Principal Proposed Uses

Diabetes

Widely sold in Asian groceries as food, bitter melon is also a folk remedy for diabetes, cancer, and various infections.

What Is Bitter Melon Used for Today?

Preliminary studies appear to confirm the first of these folk uses, suggesting that bitter melon may improve blood sugar control in people with diabetes.[1,2] If you have diabetes, you might consider adding bitter melon to your diet, but only under a doctor's supervision (see Safety Issues). (For more information on bitter melon and diabetes, see *The Natural Pharmacist Guide to Diabetes.*)

Bitter melon has also been suggested as a treatment for AIDS, but the evidence thus far is too weak to even mention. There is absolutely no evidence that it can treat cancer.

Dosage

The proper dosage is one small, unripe, raw melon or about 50 ml of fresh juice, each taken in 2 or 3 doses over the course of the day. The only problem is that bitter melon tastes *extremely* bitter. Noted naturopath Michael Murray suggests that you should "simply plug your nose and take a 2-ounce shot."[3]

Tinctures of bitter melon have begun to arrive on the market, which may make the herb a bit easier to swallow. Follow the directions on the label for correct dosage.

Safety Issues

As a widely eaten food in Asia, bitter melon is generally regarded as safe. It can cause diarrhea and stomach pain if taken in excessive amounts, but the main risk of bitter melon comes from the fact that it may work! Combining it with standard drugs may reduce blood sugar too well, possibly leading to dangerously low levels. For this reason, if you already take drugs for diabetes, you should add bitter melon to your diet only with a physician's supervision. And definitely don't stop your medication and substitute bitter melon instead! It is not as powerful as insulin or other conventional treatments.

Safety in young children, pregnant or nursing women, or those with severe liver or kidney disease has not been established.

BLACK COHOSH

(CIMICIFUGA RACEMOSA)

Principal Proposed Uses

Menopausal symptoms

Other Proposed Uses

PMS, dysmenorrhea (painful menstruation)

Black cohosh is a tall perennial herb originally found in the northeastern United States. Native Americans used it primarily for women's health problems, but also as a treatment for arthritis, fatigue, and snakebite. European colonists rapidly adopted the herb for similar uses, and in the late nineteenth century, black cohosh was the principal ingredient in the wildly popular Lydia E. Pinkham's Vegetable Compound for menstrual cramps. Migrating across the Atlantic, black cohosh became a popular European treatment for women's problems, arthritis, and high blood pressure.

What Is Black Cohosh Used for Today?

Modern German research has found that black cohosh extracts can mimic many of the effects of estrogen. In particular, the herb appears to inhibit the pituitary hormone LH, which rises to sky-high levels in menopause.[1,2,3]

Black cohosh has been approved by Germany's Commission E for use in treating menopause, dysmenorrhea, and PMS. According to the results of studies, menopausal women report distinct improvements in hot flashes, sweating, headache, vertigo, heart palpitations, tinnitus, nervousness, irritability, sleep disturbance, anxiety, and depression. (For more information on menopause, see *The Natural Pharmacist Guide to Menopause*.) Black cohosh takes 4 to 6 weeks to produce its full benefits.

Unfortunately, there is no evidence that black cohosh can prevent osteoporosis or heart disease, two of estrogen's most famous benefits.

Black cohosh appears to be only mildly effective (if at all) for treating PMS and dysmenorrhea. (For more information on PMS, see *The Natural Pharmacist Guide to PMS*.)

What Is the Scientific Evidence for Black Cohosh?

In an open study of 629 women, standardized black cohosh extract produced significant results in approximately 80% of them.[4] However, these results are made less impressive by the fact that placebo significantly reduces menopausal symptoms in about 50% of cases.[5]

Another open study of black cohosh documented actual improvements in the cells of the vaginal wall.[6] Could the placebo effect produce changes seen by microscope? Perhaps, but it seems unlikely.

The best evidence comes from a double-blind study that followed 80 women for 12 weeks, comparing the benefits of black cohosh, conjugated estrogens (0.625 mg), and placebo.[7] According to the reported results, black cohosh was actually more effective than estrogen both in relieving symptoms and in normalizing the appearance of vaginal cells under microscopic evaluation.

However, a recent double-blind study that evaluated two different dosages of black cohosh did not find any change in vaginal-cell appearance or indeed any other objective measurements that would indicate an estrogen-like effect.[8] This surprising, negative outcome was tersely reported in the product literature of one of the major manufacturers of black cohosh. Considering all the other research evidence, and the lack of detailed information about this study, I would tend to believe the earlier information instead at this time.

Dosage

The standard dosage of black cohosh is 1 or 2 tablets twice a day of a standardized extract, manufactured to contain 1 mg of 27-deoxyacteine per tablet.

Make sure not to confuse black cohosh with blue cohosh *(Caulophyllum thalictroides)*. Blue cohosh is potentially more dangerous since it contains chemicals that are toxic to the heart; a recent case report indicates that this similarly named herb caused severe heart problems in a pregnant mother.[9]

Safety Issues

Black cohosh seldom produces any side effects other than occasional mild gastrointestinal distress. Studies in rats have found no significant toxicity when black cohosh was given at 90 times the therapeutic dosage for a period of 6 months.[10] Since 6 months in a rat corresponds to decades in a human, this study appears to make a strong statement about the long-term safety of black cohosh.

Unlike estrogen, black cohosh does not stimulate breast-cancer cells growing in a test tube.[11] However, black cohosh has not yet been subjected to large-scale studies similar to those conducted for estrogen. For this reason, safety for those with previous breast cancer is not known. Also, because of hormonal activity, black cohosh is not recommended for adolescents or pregnant or nursing women.

Black cohosh has been found to slightly lower blood pressure and blood sugar in certain animals.[12] For this reason, it's possible that the herb could interact with drugs for high blood pressure or diabetes, although there are no reports of any such problems. Combination treatment with other hormonally active substances may also produce unpredictable results.

Safety in young children, or those with severe liver or kidney disease is not known.

Combining Black Cohosh with Estrogen-Replacement Therapy

Some women choose to take extremely low doses of estrogen (in the 0.312 mg range), hoping to somewhat alleviate the risk of osteoporosis without increasing the potential for breast cancer. Although there are no studies to tell us whether this will work, it is certainly a logical idea, and some gynecologists endorse it.

However, such a low dose of estrogen may not completely stop symptoms such as hot flashes. Black cohosh has been suggested as an addition to improve symptom control. While this technique has not been studied, it is again a logical idea that is probably safe (but don't ask me to guarantee it!).

Transitioning from Estrogen-Replacement Therapy to Black Cohosh

Each woman is unique but, in general, many women successfully switch over from 0.625 mg of daily estrogen to the standard dosage of black cohosh without developing symptoms. However, transitioning from higher dosages of estrogen will frequently result in breakthrough hot flashes and other symptoms. Again, remember that black cohosh is not known to offer protection against cardiovascular disease and osteoporosis.

BLOODROOT
(SANGUINARIA CANADENSIS)

Principal Proposed Uses

Oral uses: Periodontal disease prevention (used as a toothpaste or mouthwash)

Topical uses: Warts

Internal uses: Respiratory illnesses

Bloodroot is a perennial flowering herb that was widely used by Native Americans both as a reddish-orange dye and as a medicine. Some tribes drank bloodroot tea as a treatment for sore throats, fevers, and joint pain, while others applied the somewhat caustic sap to skin cancers. European herbalists used bloodroot to treat respiratory infections, asthma, joint pain, warts, ringworm, and nasal polyps.

In the mid 1800s, a Dr. Fells of Middlesex Hospital in London developed a cancer treatment consisting of a paste of bloodroot, flour, water, and zinc chloride applied directly to breast tumors and other cancers. Similar formulations were used in various locales up through the turn of the century. Bloodroot was a common constituent of "drawing salves" believed capable of "pulling" tumors out of the body.

What Is Bloodroot Used for Today?

Herbalists frequently recommend bloodroot pastes and salves for the treatment of warts. Bloodroot is an *escharotic,* that is to say a scab-producing substance, and it functions much like commercial wart plasters containing salicylic acid. Although there has not been any real scientific study of the use of bloodroot for warts, based on its immediate effects it is likely to help at least somewhat.

One constituent of bloodroot, sanguinarine, appears to possess topical antibiotic properties.[1] On this basis, the FDA has approved the use of bloodroot in commercially available toothpastes and oral rinses to inhibit the development of dental plaque and periodontal disease (gingivitis).

Bloodroot is also often combined with other herbs in cough syrups. Some herbalists recommend drinking bloodroot tea for respiratory ailments, but others consider the herb to be too unpredictable in its side effects.

While scientific research has found constituents in bloodroot that possess antitumor properties,[2] there is no evidence that the herb can cure cancer. Undoubtedly bloodroot pastes can nibble away at tumors the same way they dissolve warts. However, such an approach is not likely to cure a malignant tumor, and might actually spread it.

Dosage

For the treatment of warts, bloodroot can be made into a paste and applied directly to the involved area. However, start slowly to see how sensitive you are. Excessive application can lead to severe burns. Once you've discovered your tolerance, apply the herb for a day or so, then remove it and wait for the scab to develop and then drop off. This process can be repeated until the wart is gone.

Bloodroot tea for treating respiratory illnesses may be made by boiling 1 teaspoon of powdered root in a cup of water and taken 2 or 3 times daily.

Safety Issues

Oral bloodroot appears to be relatively safe and nontoxic.[3] However, in large doses, it causes nausea and vomiting, and even at lower dosages it has been known to cause peculiar side effects in some people, such as tunnel vision and pain in the feet. For this reason, many herbalists recommend that it be used only under the supervision of a qualified practitioner.

Topical applications of bloodroot can cause severe burns if used too vigorously and for too long a time. Safety in young children, pregnant or nursing women, or those with severe liver or kidney disease is not established.

BOSWELLIA

(BOSWELLIA SERRATA)

Principal Proposed Uses

Rheumatoid arthritis, osteoarthritis, bursitis, tendinitis

The gummy resin of the boswellia tree has a long history of use in Indian herbal medicine as a treatment for arthritis, bursitis, respiratory diseases, and diarrhea.

What Is Boswellia Used for Today?

Boswellia is often recommended as a treatment for arthritis (both osteo- and rheumatoid), bursitis, and tendinitis, based on the recent work of Indian scientists. Investigations of boswellia have shown that the herb contains certain substances known as *boswellic acids*, which appear to possess anti-inflammatory properties.[1,2] Other preliminary research suggests that boswellia may improve the biochemical structure of cartilage.[3] (For more information on arthritis, see *The Natural Pharmacist Guide to Arthritis*.)

What Is the Scientific Evidence for Boswellia?

According to a recent review of unpublished studies, preliminary double-blind trials have found boswellia effective in rheumatoid arthritis.[4] Two placebo-controlled studies, involving a total of 81 individuals with rheumatoid arthritis, found significant reductions in swelling and pain over the course of 3 months.

Also, a comparative study of 60 people over 6 months found that boswellia extract produced symptomatic benefits comparable to oral gold therapy. However, this review was rather sketchy on details. It did not state whether or not boswellia could induce remission like gold shots, and not enough information was given to evaluate the quality of the research.

However, a recent double-blind placebo-controlled study that enrolled 78 patients found no benefit.[5] About half of the patients dropped out, which diminishes the significance of the results.

There has not been any formal study of boswellia's effectiveness in osteoarthritis.

Dosage

A typical dose of boswellia is 400 mg 3 times a day of an extract standardized to contain 37.5% boswellic acids. The full effect may take 4 to 8 weeks to develop.

Safety Issues

Although comprehensive safety testing has not been completed, boswellia appears to be reasonably safe when used as directed. Side effects are rare and consist primarily of occasional allergic reactions or mild gastrointestinal distress. Safety in young children, pregnant or nursing women, or those with severe liver or kidney disease is not established.

BROMELAIN
(PINEAPPLE STEM)

Principal Proposed Uses

Reducing swelling and inflammation (e.g., recovery after surgery or athletic injuries, vein inflammation, arthritis, dysmenorrhea)

Digestive problems (e.g., "weak" digestion, food allergies)

Bromelain is not actually a single substance, but rather a collection of protein-digesting enzymes found in pineapple juice and in the stem of pineapple plants. It is primarily produced in Japan, Hawaii, and Taiwan, and much of the original research was performed in the first two of those locations. Subsequently, European researchers developed an interest, and by 1995 bromelain had become the thirteenth most common individual herbal product sold in Germany.

What Is Bromelain Used for Today?

In 1993, Germany's Commission E approved bromelain for "reducing swelling in the nose and sinuses caused by injuries and operations." The reason for this narrow recommendation is that when the commissioners reviewed the available evidence the only reliable studies they could find involved these specific conditions. However, bromelain is actually thought to be useful for other conditions as well, based on its apparent ability to reduce swelling and inflammation. In Europe, bromelain is widely used to aid in recovery from surgery and athletic injuries, as well as to treat diseases of veins, arthritis, and menstrual pain (dysmenorrhea).

Bromelain is also useful as a digestive enzyme. Unlike most digestive enzymes, bromelain is active both in the acid environment of the stomach and the alkaline environment of the small intestine.[1,2] This may make it particularly effective as an oral digestive aid for those who do not digest proteins properly. Since it is primarily the proteins in foods that cause food allergies, bromelain might reduce food-allergy symptoms as well, although this has not been proven.

What Is the Scientific Evidence for Bromelain?

While most large enzymes are broken down in the digestive tract, those found in bromelain appear to be absorbed whole to a certain extent.[3] This finding makes it reasonable to suppose that bromelain can actually produce systemic (whole body) effects. Once in the blood, bromelain appears to produce mild anti-inflammatory and "blood-thinning" effects.[4-7]

In 1993, Germany's Commission E reviewed the evidence for bromelain's effectiveness in reducing the swelling caused by injury or surgery. They found five passable double-blind studies, of which three showed good results and two showed no benefit.[8] In their opinion, the best evidence was for swelling in the nose and sinuses.

Another double-blind study followed 73 people being treated for phlebitis, or inflammation of the veins of the leg.[9] Those who received bromelain in addition to standard treatments showed improved results.

Warning: Do not attempt to self-treat phlebitis.

An open study of 146 boxers suggested that bromelain helps bruises to heal more quickly.[10]

Dosage

A typical dosage of bromelain is 500 mg 3 times daily between meals, or with meals for use as a digestive aid.

The strength of bromelain is measured in MCUs (milk-clotting units). A good preparation should contain 2,000 MCUs per gram.

Safety Issues

Bromelain appears to be essentially nontoxic, and it seldom causes side effects other than occasional mild gastrointestinal distress or allergic reactions.[11]

However, because bromelain "thins the blood" to some extent, it shouldn't be combined with drugs such as Coumadin (warfarin) without a doctor's supervision.

Safety in young children, pregnant or nursing women, or those with liver or kidney disease has not been established.

BURDOCK
(ARCTIUM LAPPA)

Principal Proposed Uses

Eczema, psoriasis, acne

Other Proposed Uses

Cancer?

The common burdock, that well-known source of annoying burrs matted in dogs' fur, is also a medicinal herb of considerable reputation. Called *gobo* in Japan, burdock root is said to be a food that provides deep strengthening to the immune system. In ancient China and India, herbalists used it in the treatment of respiratory infections, abscesses, and joint pain. European physicians of the Middle Ages and later used it to treat cancerous tumors, skin conditions, venereal disease, and bladder and kidney problems.

Burdock was a primary ingredient in the famous (or infamous) Hoxsey cancer treatment. Harry Hoxsey was a former coal miner who parlayed a traditional family remedy for cancer into the largest privately owned cancer treatment center in the world, with branches in 17 states. (It was shut down in the 1950s by the FDA. Harry Hoxsey himself subsequently died of cancer.) Other herbs in his formula included red clover, poke, prickly ash, bloodroot, and barberry. Burdock is also found in the famous herbal cancer remedy Essiac.

Despite this historical enthusiasm, there is no significant evidence that burdock is an effective treatment for cancer or any other illness.

What Is Burdock Used for Today?

Burdock is widely recommended for the relief of dry, scaly skin conditions such as eczema and psoriasis. It is also used for treating acne. It can be taken internally as well as applied directly to the skin. Unfortunately, there is no real scientific evidence for any of these uses.

Dosage

A typical dosage of burdock is 1 to 2 g of powdered dry root 3 times per day.

Safety Issues

As a food commonly eaten in Japan (it is often found in sukiyaki), burdock root is believed to be safe. However, in 1978, the *Journal of the American Medical Association* caused a brief scare by publishing a report of burdock poisoning. Subsequent investigation showed that the herbal product involved was actually contaminated with the poisonous chemical atropine from an unknown source.[1] Safety in young children, pregnant or nursing women, or those with severe liver or kidney disease is not established.

BUTCHER'S BROOM
(RUSCUS ACULEATUS)

Principal Proposed Uses
Hemorrhoids, varicose veins

So-named because its branches were a traditional source of broom straw used by butchers, this Mediterranean evergreen bush has a long history of traditional use in the treatment of urinary conditions.

What Is Butcher's Broom Used for Today?

Butcher's broom has been approved by Germany's Commission E as supportive therapy for hemorrhoids and varicose veins.

Preliminary evidence from animal studies suggests that butcher's broom possesses anti-inflammatory properties and also constricts small veins.[1,2] Double-blind studies in people have not yet been reported.

Dosage

Butcher's broom is standardized to its *ruscogenin* content. A typical oral dose should supply 50 to 100 mg of ruscogenins daily.

For hemorrhoids, butcher's broom can also be applied as an ointment or in the form of a suppository.

Safety Issues

Butcher's broom is believed to be safe when used as directed, although detailed studies have not been performed. Noticeable side effects are rare. Safety in young children, pregnant or nursing women, or those with liver or kidney disease has not been established.

CALENDULA a.k.a. MARIGOLD

(CALENDULA OFFICINALIS)

Principal Proposed Uses

Topical uses: Skin injuries (e.g., cuts, scrapes, burns, nonhealing wounds), skin inflammation (e.g., eczema), hemorrhoids, varicose veins

Oral uses: Mouth sores

Calendula, well known as one of the ornamental marigolds, blooms month after month from early spring to first frost. Because "calend" means month in Latin, the plant's lengthy flowering season is believed to have given calendula its name. The herb has been used to heal wounds and treat inflamed skin since ancient times.

An active ingredient that might be responsible for calendula's traditional medicinal properties has not been discovered. One theory suggests that volatile oils in the plant act synergistically with other constituents called *xanthophylls*.[1]

What Is Calendula Used for Today?

Experiments on rats and other animals suggest that calendula cream exerts a wound-healing and anti-inflammatory effect,[2,3] but double-blind studies have not yet been reported.

Creams made with calendula flower are a nearly ubiquitous item in the German medicine chest, used for everything from children's scrapes to eczema, burns, and poorly healing wounds. These same German products are widely available in the United States as well.

Calendula cream is also used to soothe hemorrhoids and varicose veins, and the tea reportedly reduces the discomfort of mouth sores.

According to Germany's Commission E, calendula can also be taken as a tea for inflammatory conditions of the mouth.

Dosage

Calendula cream should be applied 2 or 3 times daily to the affected area. For oral use as a mouthwash, pour boiling water over 1 to 2 teaspoons of calendula flowers and allow to steep for 10 to 15 minutes. Rinse your mouth with this liquid several times a day.

Safety Issues

Calendula is generally regarded as safe. Neither calendula cream nor calendula taken internally has been associated with any adverse effects other than occasional allergic reactions.

CAT'S CLAW

(UNCARIA TOMENTOSA)

Principal Proposed Uses

Various viral diseases (genital and oral herpes, shingles [herpes zoster], AIDS, feline leukemia virus), allergies, arthritis, ulcers

---

Cat's claw is a popular herb among the indigenous people of Peru, where it is used to treat cancer, diabetes, ulcers, arthritis, and infections, as well as assist in recovery from childbirth. It is also used as a contraceptive.

Scientific studies of cat's claw conducted in Peru, Italy, Austria, and Germany have yielded numerous intriguing findings, but as yet no conclusive proof of any healing benefit. Nonetheless, with increasing international popularity, cultivation of cat's claw has become a major revenue source for the Ashaninka Indian tribe of Peru.

What Is Cat's Claw Used for Today?

In Europe and Peru, cat's claw is considered a promising treatment for viral diseases such as herpes, shingles, AIDS, and feline leukemia virus. Its possible use for treating allergies, stomach ulcers, and arthritis is also being studied.[1] However, the best description of the present state of affairs is that we don't yet know whether cat's claw really works. It certainly is not a proven treatment for cancer.

Dosage

The optimum dosage of cat's claw is not clear. Because of the wide variation in the forms and preparations sold, I recommend following the directions on the product's label.

Safety Issues

There have not been any reports of serious adverse effects from taking cat's claw. However, European physicians believe that it should not be taken in conjunction with hormone treatments, insulin, or vaccines.[2] Safety in young children, pregnant or nursing women, or those with severe liver or kidney disease is not established.

CAYENNE
(CAPSICUM FRUTESCENS, CAPSICUM ANNUUM)

Principal Proposed Uses

Topical uses: Post-herpetic neuralgia, arthritis, and other forms of pain

Oral uses: Heart disease

The capsicum family includes red peppers, bell peppers, pimento, and paprika, but the most famous medicinal member of this family is the common cayenne pepper. The substance capsaicin is the common "hot" ingredient in all hot peppers.

Cayenne and related peppers have a long history of use as digestive aids in many parts of the world, but the herb's recent popularity has, surprisingly, come through conventional medicine.

What Is Cayenne Used for Today?

Under the brand name Zostrix, a cream containing concentrated capsaicin has been approved by the FDA for the treatment of the pain that often lingers after an attack of shingles (technically, post-herpetic neuralgia). There is also some evidence that capsaicin creams may be helpful for relieving arthritis as well as other forms of pain.

Cayenne pepper taken internally has recently been widely touted as a treatment for heart disease by those who have found it useful for themselves or others, but there is no scientific evidence that it is effective.

Dosage

Capsaicin creams are approved over-the-counter drugs and should be used as directed.

For internal use, cayenne may be taken at a dosage of 1 to 2 standard 00 gelatin capsules 1 to 3 times daily.

Safety Issues

As a commonly used food, cayenne is generally regarded as safe. Contrary to some reports, cayenne does not appear to aggravate stomach ulcers.[1]

CHAMOMILE

GERMAN (MATRICARIA RECUTITA); ROMAN (CHAMAEMELUM NOBILE)

Principal Proposed Uses

Topical uses: Skin inflammation (e.g., dermatitis and eczema), wound healing

Oral uses: Gastrointestinal discomfort, anxiety, insomnia, arthritis, asthma

Two distinct plants are known as chamomile and are used interchangeably: German and Roman chamomile. Although botanically far apart, they both look like miniature daisies and appear to possess similar medicinal benefits.

Over a million cups of chamomile tea are drunk daily, testifying to its good taste and fine reputation. Chamomile was used by early Egyptian physicians for fevers and by ancient Greeks, Romans, and Indians for headaches and disorders of the kidneys, liver, and bladder. Modern-day Germans employ it for digestive upsets and menstrual difficulties, and the British use it for all these purposes.

It has been suggested that chamomile's reported effect is due to the constituents of its bright blue oil, including chamazulene, alpha-bisabolol, and bisaboloxides. However, the water-soluble part of chamomile may play a role, too, especially in soothing stomach upset.

What Is Chamomile Used for Today?

The modern use of chamomile dates back to 1921, when a German firm introduced a topical form of chamomile named Kamillosan. This cream became a popular treatment for a wide variety of skin disorders, including eczema, bedsores, post-radiation therapy skin inflammation, and contact dermatitis (e.g., poison ivy).

Chamomile tea is widely used as a folk remedy to soothe colicky pains in the digestive tract and help induce sleep. Concentrated alcohol extracts of chamomile are also sometimes used to treat arthritis pain. (For more information on arthritis, see *The Natural Pharmacist Guide to Arthritis.*) Finally, it is common practice in Germany for individuals with asthma or other breathing problems to inhale the steam from boiling chamomile and other herbs.

What Is the Scientific Evidence for Chamomile?

Numerous case reports and controlled (but not blinded) studies have consistently found significant benefits of chamomile cream in inflammatory skin diseases and wound healing.[1]

Animal research suggests that chamomile extracts taken orally can relax the intestines and reduce inflammation.[2] However, properly performed double-blind studies are lacking.

Dosage

Chamomile cream is applied to the affected area 1 to 4 times daily.

Chamomile tea can be made by pouring boiling water over 2 to 3 heaping teaspoons of flowers and steeping for 10 minutes.

Chamomile tinctures and pills should be taken according to the directions on the label. Alcoholic tincture may be the most potent form for internal use.

Safety Issues

Chamomile is listed on the FDA's GRAS (generally regarded as safe) list.

Reports that chamomile can cause severe reactions in people allergic to ragweed have received significant media attention. However, when all the evidence is examined, it does not appear that chamomile is actually more allergenic than any other plant.[3] The cause of these reports may be product contaminated with "dog chamomile," a highly allergenic and bad-tasting plant of similar appearance.

Chamomile also contains naturally occurring coumarin compounds that can act as "blood thinners." Excessive use of chamomile is therefore not recommended when taking prescription anticoagulants.

Safety in young children, pregnant or nursing women, or those with liver or kidney disease has not been established, although there have not been any credible reports of toxicity caused by this common beverage tea.

CHASTEBERRY

(VITEX AGNUS-CASTUS)

Principal Proposed Uses

Cyclic breast discomfort (often associated with PMS), other PMS symptoms, menstrual irregularities, female infertility

Other Proposed Uses

Menopausal symptoms

Chasteberry is frequently called by its Latin names: *vitex* or, alternatively, *agnus-castus*. A shrub in the verbena family, chasteberry is commonly found on riverbanks and nearby foothills in central Asia and around the Mediterranean Sea. After its violet flowers have bloomed, a dark brown, peppercorn-size fruit, with a pleasant odor reminiscent of peppermint, develops. This fruit is used medicinally.

As the name implies, for centuries chasteberry was thought to counter sexual desire. A drink prepared from the plant's seeds was used by the Romans to diminish libido, and in ancient Greece, young women celebrating the festival of Demeter wore chasteberry blossoms to show that they were remaining chaste in honor of the goddess. Monks in the Middle Ages used the fruit for similar purposes, yielding the common name "monk's pepper."

What Is Chasteberry Used for Today?

The modern use of chasteberry dates back to the 1950s, when the German pharmaceutical firm Madaus Company first produced a standardized extract. This herb has become a standard European treatment for the cyclical breast tenderness that is often associated with PMS, which is sometimes called *cyclic mastitis, cyclic mastalgia, mastodynia,* or *fibrocystic breast disease.* Chasteberry is also used for general PMS symptoms, as well as menstrual irregularities and infertility. The herb's full benefits are believed to take several months to develop, so be patient.

Research has shown that, unlike other herbs used for women's health problems, chasteberry does not contain any plant equivalent of estrogen or progesterone. Rather, it acts on the pituitary gland to suppress the release of prolactin.[1-4] Prolactin is a hormone that naturally rises during pregnancy to stimulate milk production. Inappropriately increased production of prolactin may be a factor in cyclic breast tenderness, as well as other symptoms of PMS. Elevated prolactin levels can also cause a woman's period to become irregular and even stop. For this reason, chasteberry is often tried for irregular or absent menstrual flow. However, I recommend that you do not attempt to self-treat significant menstrual irregularities without a full medical evaluation. There could be a serious medical condition causing the problem that you wouldn't want to miss.

High prolactin levels can also cause infertility. For this reason, chasteberry is sometimes tried as a fertility drug.[5]

Finally, chasteberry occasionally appears to be dramatically effective at reducing menopausal symptoms. Strangely, it is just as often totally ineffective.

What Is the Scientific Evidence for Chasteberry?

Despite its widespread use in Germany, the scientific record for chasteberry is not as strong as it should be.

Premenstrual Syndrome

German gynecologists clearly believe that chasteberry is effective for PMS. In a rather informal study enrolling more than 1,500 women with PMS, doctors rated chasteberry as effective about 90% of the time.[6,7] Women reported significant or complete improvement in such symptoms as breast pain, fluid retention, headache, and fatigue.

However, this study did not involve a placebo group, and all the patients knew they were being treated. It is impossible to tell from the results what fraction of the benefit was due to the power of suggestion alone. It is a known fact that placebo treatment is highly effective for PMS, often reducing symptoms by as much as 70%.[8] Thus, the results of this study are more a survey of physicians' experiences with chasteberry than actual scientific evidence.

The opinion of experienced physicians is meaningful, but it's definitely not proof. Decades of experience have shown us how easy it is for even seasoned professionals to over- or underestimate the effectiveness of a treatment, based on their preconceptions and the power of suggestion. When it comes to medical treatments, well-designed scientific studies are required to produce dependable evidence.

However, a search of medical literature conducted during the writing of this book failed to find any double-blind placebo-controlled studies that directly evaluated the benefits of chasteberry for PMS symptoms. One double-blind study has been performed, but unfortunately it compared chasteberry to vitamin B_6 (pyridoxine) instead of a placebo.[9]

Published in 1997, this study followed 175 women who were given either a standardized chasteberry extract or 200 mg of vitamin B_6 daily. Chasteberry proved to be at least as effective as vitamin B_6. Both treatments produced significant improvements in all major symptoms of PMS, including breast tenderness, edema, tension, headache, and depression.

Although this study has been widely described as evidence that chasteberry is effective for PMS, it doesn't actually prove anything at all. Vitamin B_6 itself has not been proven effective for PMS.[10] Therefore, the fact that chasteberry works just as well as vitamin B_6 establishes little! It is quite possible that much of the improvement seen in both groups was due to the placebo effect. We really need a good, large-scale, double-blind placebo-controlled study to discover just how effective chasteberry is, beyond the inevitable effects of suggestion. (For more information on PMS, see *The Natural Pharmacist Guide to PMS.*)

Irregular Menstruation

One double-blind trial followed 52 women with a form of irregular menstruation known as *luteal phase defect*.[11] This condition is believed to be related to excessive prolactin release. After 3 months, the women who took chasteberry showed significant improvements.

Dosage

There are many different types of chasteberry preparations on the market. Each should be taken according to its label instruction.

Safety Issues

There haven't been any detailed studies of the safety of chasteberry. However, its widespread use in Germany has not led to any reports of significant adverse effects,[12] other than a single case of excessive ovarian stimulation possibly caused by chasteberry.[13]

Because it lowers prolactin levels, chasteberry is not an appropriate treatment for pregnant or nursing women. Safety in young children or those with severe liver or kidney disease has not been established.

There are no known drug interactions associated with chasteberry. However, it is quite conceivable that the herb could interfere with other hormonal medications, such as birth control pills.

COLEUS FORSKOHLII

Principal Proposed Uses

Allergic conditions (e.g., asthma, eczema, allergies)

Muscle contraction (e.g., asthma, high blood pressure, menstrual cramps, irritable bowel [spastic colon], bladder pain, glaucoma)

Other Proposed Uses

Psoriasis

A member of the mint family, *Coleus forskohlii* grows wild on the mountain slopes of Nepal, India, and Thailand. In traditional Asian systems of medicine, it was used for a variety of purposes, including treating skin rashes, asthma, bronchitis, insomnia, epilepsy, and angina. But modern interest is based almost entirely on the work of a drug company, Hoechst Pharmaceuticals.

Like other drug manufacturers, Hoechst regularly screens medicinal plants in hopes of discovering new medications. In 1974, work performed in collaboration with the Indian Central Drug Research Institute found that the rootstalk of *Coleus forskohlii* could lower blood pressure and decrease muscle spasms. Intensive study identified a substance named forskolin that appeared to be responsible for much of this effect.

Forskolin is a substance with unique biological activity. It increases the levels of a fundamental natural compound known as *cyclic AMP*.[1,2] Cyclic AMP plays a major role in an immense variety of cellular functions, and, by altering its levels, forskolin has the ability to profoundly alter many aspects of body functioning. Forskolin and synthetic substances patterned after it may eventually form an entirely new class of drugs.

Yet, while all this information about forskolin is interesting, it does not necessarily say anything about the effects of the whole herb itself.

What Is *Coleus forskohlii* Used for Today?

Herb manufacturers have begun to offer extracts of *Coleus forskohlii* that have been specially manufactured to contain high levels of forskolin.

Forskolin has been found to stabilize the cells that release histamine and other inflammatory compounds.[3] This suggests that *Coleus forskohlii* may be a useful treatment for asthma, eczema, and other allergic conditions.

Studies have also found that forskolin relaxes smooth muscle tissue.[4,5] For this reason, *Coleus forskohlii* has been suggested as a treatment for asthma, menstrual cramps, irritable bowel syndrome (spastic colon), crampy bladder pain (as in bladder infections), and high blood pressure.

Coleus forskohlii has also been proposed as a treatment for psoriasis, because that disease appears to be at least partly related to low levels of cyclic AMP in skin cells.

What Is the Scientific Evidence for *Coleus forskohlii?*

The scientific evidence for the herb *Coleus forskohlii* as a treatment for any disease is weak. What is known relates to the substance forskolin rather than the whole herb.

Animal studies and open studies in humans suggest that forskolin can reduce blood pressure and dilate bronchial tubes.[6,7,8] A tiny double-blind study indicates that forskolin taken by inhalation may be as effective as standard asthma inhalers,[9] and forskolin eye drops appear to improve glaucoma.[10]

Dosage

A common dosage recommendation is 50 mg 2 or 3 times a day of an extract standardized to contain 18% forskolin.

However, because such an extract provides significant levels of forskolin, a drug with wide-ranging properties, I recommend that *Coleus forskohlii* extracts should be taken only with a doctor's supervision.

Safety Issues

The safety of *Coleus forskohlii* and forskolin has not been fully evaluated, although few significant risks have been noted in studies performed thus far. Caution should be exercised when combining this herb with blood-pressure medications and "blood thinners." Safety in young children, pregnant or nursing women, or those with severe liver or kidney disease has not been established.

CRANBERRY
(VACCINIUM MACROCARPON)

Principal Proposed Uses

Bladder infections (prevention and possible treatment)

The cranberry plant is a close relative of the common blueberry. Native Americans used it both as food and for the treatment of bladder and kidney diseases. The Pilgrims learned about cranberry from local tribes, and quickly adopted it for their own use. Subsequent physicians used it for bladder infections, for "bladder gravel" (small bladder stones), and to remove "blood toxins."

In the 1920s, researchers observed that drinking cranberry juice makes the urine more acidic. Since common urinary tract–infection bacteria such as *E. coli* dislike acidic surroundings, physicians concluded that they had discovered a scientific explanation for the traditional uses of cranberry. This discovery led to widespread medical use of cranberry juice for treating bladder infections. Cranberry fell out of favor with physicians after World War II, but it became popular again during the 1960s—as a self-treatment.

What Is Cranberry Used for Today?

Cranberry is widely used today to prevent bladder infections. Contrary to the research from the 1920s, it now appears that acidification of the urine is not so important as cranberry's ability to block bacteria from adhering to the bladder wall.[1,2,3] If the bacteria can't hold on they will be washed out with the stream of urine.

Cranberry juice is believed to be most effective as a form of prevention. When taken regularly, it appears to reduce the frequency of recurrent bladder infections in women prone to develop them. Cranberry may also be helpful during a bladder infection but not as reliably.

What Is the Scientific Evidence for Cranberry?

Most of the clinical research about cranberry has involved elderly women. The largest study followed 153 women with an average age of 78.5 years for a period of 6 months.[4] Half were given a standard commercial cranberry cocktail drink, the other a placebo drink prepared to look and taste the same. Both treatments contained the same amount of vitamin C to eliminate the possible antibacterial influence of that supplement.

Despite the weak preparation of cranberry used, the results showed a 58% decrease in the incidence of bacteria and white blood cells in the urine.

Interestingly, studies have found that in women who develop frequent bladder infections, bacteria seem to have a particularly easy time holding on to the bladder wall.[5] This suggests that cranberry juice can actually get to the root of their problem, but more research is needed.

Dosage

The proper dosage of dry cranberry juice extract is 300 to 400 mg twice daily. For people who prefer juice, 8 to 16 ounces daily should suffice. Pure cranberry juice and not sugary cranberry juice cocktail with its low percentage of cranberry should be used for best effect.

Safety Issues

There are no known risks of this food for adults, children, or pregnant or nursing women. However, cranberry juice may allow the kidneys to excrete certain drugs more rapidly, thereby reducing their effectiveness. All weakly alkaline drugs may be affected, including many antidepressants and prescription painkillers.

DAMIANA
(TURNERA DIFFUSA)

Principal Proposed Uses

Male sexual capacity

Other Proposed Uses

Respiratory diseases (e.g., asthma), depression, digestive problems, sexual dysfunction, menstrual disorders

---

The herb damiana has been used in Mexico for some time as a male aphrodisiac.[1] Classic herbal literature of the nineteenth century describes it as a "tonic," or general body strengthener.

What Is Damiana Used for Today?

Damiana continues to be a popular aphrodisiac for males. However, if it works at all, the effect appears to be rather mild. No scientific trials have been reported.

Damiana is also sometimes said to be helpful for treating asthma and other respiratory diseases, depression, digestive problems, various forms of sexual dysfunction, and menstrual disorders.[2,3]

Like the herb uva ursi, damiana contains arbutin, although at a concentration about 10 times lower. Arbutin is a urinary antiseptic, but the levels present in damiana are probably too small to make this herb a useful treatment for bladder infections.

Dosage

The proper dosage of damiana is 2 to 4 g taken 2 to 3 times daily, or as directed on the label.

Safety Issues

Damiana appears to be safe at the recommended dosages. It appears on the FDA's GRAS list and is widely used as a food flavoring. However, because damiana contains low levels of cyanide-like compounds, excessive doses may be dangerous. Safety in young children, pregnant or nursing women, or those with severe liver or kidney disease is not established. The only common side effect of damiana is occasional mild gastrointestinal distress.

DANDELION

(TARAXACUM OFFICINALE)

Principal Proposed Uses

Fluid retention (leaves), nutritional supplement (leaves), liver/gallbladder disease (root)

The common dandelion, enemy of suburban lawns, is an unusually nutritious food. Its leaves contain substantial levels of vitamins A, C, D, and B complex, as well as iron, magnesium, zinc, potassium, manganese, copper, choline, calcium, boron, and silicon.

Worldwide, the root of the dandelion has been used for the treatment of a variety of liver and gallbladder problems. Other historical uses of the root and leaves include the treatment of breast diseases, water retention, digestive problems, joint pain, fever, and skin diseases. The most active constituents in dandelion appear to be eudesmanolide and germacranolide, substances unique to this herb.

What Is Dandelion Used for Today?

Dandelion leaves are widely recommended as a food supplement for pregnant and also postmenopausal women because of the many nutrients they contain. They also appear to produce a mild diuretic effect, which may be appreciated by those who suffer from fluid retention.

Based on tradition, herbalists frequently suggest dandelion root for liver diseases. However, exactly which liver disease dandelion may be useful for and whether it simply relieves symptoms or actually helps cure the condition remains unclear.

The scientific basis for the use of dandelion is scanty. Preliminary studies suggest that dandelion root stimulates the flow of bile.[1] Dandelion leaves have also been found to produce a mild diuretic effect.[2]

Dosage

A typical dosage of dandelion root is 2 to 8 g 3 times daily. The leaves may be eaten in salad or cooked.

Safety Issues

Dandelion root and leaves are believed to be quite safe, with no side effects other than rare allergic reactions.[3] Because the leaves contain so much potassium, they probably resupply any potassium lost due to dandelion's mild diuretic effect, although this has not been proven. However, safety in young children, pregnant or nursing women, or those with severe liver or kidney disease has not been established.

DEVIL'S CLAW
(HARPAGOPHYTUM PROCUMBENS)

Principal Proposed Uses

Pain and inflammation (e.g., various types of arthritis, gout, bursitis, tendinitis)

Digestive problems (e.g., loss of appetite, mild stomach upset)

Devil's claw is a native of South Africa, so named because of its rather peculiar appearance. (An herbalist friend of mine says it looks like "an intelligent alien plant.") Its large tuberous roots are used medicinally, after being chopped up and dried in the sun for 3 days.

Native South Africans used the herb to reduce pain and fever and stimulate digestion. European colonists brought devil's claw back home, where it became a popular treatment for arthritis.

What Is Devil's Claw Used for Today?

In modern Europe, devil's claw is used to treat all types of joint pain, including osteoarthritis, rheumatoid arthritis, and gout. Devil's claw is also used for soft-tissue pain, such as bursitis and tendinitis. (For more information on arthritis, see *The Natural Pharmacist Guide to Arthritis*.)

Like other bitter herbs (and this is one of the bitterest!), devil's claw is said to improve appetite and relieve mild stomach upset.

What Is the Scientific Evidence for Devil's Claw?

One double-blind study followed 89 individuals with rheumatoid arthritis for a 2-month period. The group given devil's claw showed a significant decrease in pain intensity and improved mobility.[1]

Another double-blind study of 50 people with various types of arthritis found that 10 days of treatment with devil's claw provided significant pain relief.[2]

A recent double-blind study of 118 participants suggests that devil's claw may also help relieve soft-tissue pain (muscles, tendons, etc.).[3]

We don't know how devil's claw works. Some studies have found an anti-inflammatory effect but others have not.[4,5] Apparently, the herb doesn't produce the same changes in prostaglandins as standard anti-inflammatory drugs.[6]

Dosage

A typical dosage of devil's claw is 750 mg 3 times daily of a preparation standardized to contain 3% iridoid glycosides.

Safety Issues

Devil's claw appears to be quite safe, with no evidence of toxicity at doses many times higher than recommended.[7] A 6-month open study of 630 people with arthritis showed no side effects other than occasional mild gastrointestinal distress. However, devil's claw is not recommended for people with ulcers. Safety in young children, pregnant or nursing women, or those with severe liver or kidney disease has not been established.

DONG QUAI

(ANGELICA SINENSIS)

Principal Proposed Uses

Menstrual disorders, PMS

Probably Ineffective Uses

Menopausal symptoms (when taken alone)

One of the major herbs in the Chinese repertoire, *Angelica sinensis* is closely related to European *Angelica archangelica*, a common garden herb and the flavoring in Benedictine and Chartreuse liqueurs. The carrot-like roots of this fragrant plant are harvested in the fall after about 3 years of cultivation and stored in airtight containers prior to processing.

Traditionally, dong quai is said to be one of the most important herbs for strengthening the "xue." The Chinese term "xue" is often translated as "blood," but it actually refers to a complex concept of which the blood itself is only a part. In the late 1800s, an extract of dong quai known as *Eumenol* became popular in Europe as a "female tonic," and this is how most people still understand it in the West.

What Is Dong Quai Used for Today?

Dong quai is often recommended as a treatment for menstrual cramps and PMS, as well as hot flashes and other symptoms of menopause. The scientific evidence regarding these uses is very weak, consisting primarily of test-tube and animal studies, as well as a few uncontrolled studies of people.[1–5] Furthermore, a recent 24-week study compared the effects of dong quai against a placebo in 71 postmenopausal women.[6] According to the results, dong quai does not reduce menopausal symptoms at all.

Dong quai may be more effective when used in traditional herbal formulas. Two of the most common are Dong Quai and Paeonia, and Bupleurum and Dong Quai. These herbal combinations are frequently used for treating certain types of menopausal symptoms, as well as menstrual pain, fibrocystic breast disease, PMS, abnormal fetal movements, and pelvic inflammatory disease.[7,8,9] However, there is no scientific evidence that they are effective.

Another popular herbal formula is Dong Quai 4, so named because of the total number of herbs involved. This combination, with variations tailored to the individual, is traditionally used to treat certain forms of menstrual irregularity, menstrual pain, anemia, and insomnia.[10,11] A competent Chinese herbalist can tell you which formula would be best for you (according to tradition), as well as adjust the constituents to exactly match your personal needs.

Dosage

I recommend using dong quai under the supervision of a qualified Chinese herbalist, not because the herb is dangerous, but because it is difficult to self-prescribe Chinese herbal formulas.

If you wish to self-treat with dong quai, a typical dosage is 10 to 40 drops of dong quai tincture 1 to 3 times daily, or 1 standard 00 gelatin capsule 3 times daily.

Safety Issues

Dong quai is believed to be generally nontoxic. Very large amounts have been given to rats without causing harm.[12] Side effects are rare and primarily consist of mild gastrointestinal distress and occasional allergic reactions (such as rash).

Certain constituents of dong quai can cause increased sensitivity to the sun, but this has not been observed to occur in people using the whole herb.

According to traditional beliefs, inappropriate long-term use of dong quai (such as taking it as a single herb rather than in a combination) can damage the digestive tract and cause other disturbances in overall health. Dong quai is also generally contraindicated during the first 3 months of pregnancy and during acute respiratory infections, and in women with excessively heavy menstruation. However, there is no scientific evidence for these concerns. Safety in young children, pregnant or nursing women, or those with severe liver or kidney disease has not been established.

ECHINACEA

(ECHINACEA PURPUREA, E. ANGUSTIFOLIA, E. PALLIDA)

Principal Uses

Colds and flus (shortening the duration, reducing symptoms)

Other Possible Uses

Stimulating immunity ("aborting" a cold that has just started, reducing the number of colds during cold season, helping the body fight off other infections)

The decorative plant *Echinacea purpurea*, or purple cone-flower, has been one of the most popular herbal medications in both the United States and Europe for over a century.

Native Americans used the related species *Echinacea angustifolia* for a wide variety of problems, including respiratory infections and snakebite. Herbal physicians among the European colonists quickly added the herb to their repertoire. Echinacea became tremendously popular toward the end of the nineteenth century, when a businessman named H. C. F. Meyer promoted an herbal concoction containing *E. angustifolia*. The garish, exaggerated, and poorly written nature of his labeling helped define the characteristics of a "snake oil" remedy.

However, serious manufacturers developed an interest in echinacea as well. By 1920, the respected Lloyd Brothers Pharmaceutical company of Cincinnati, Ohio, counted echinacea as its largest selling product. In Europe, physicians took up the American interest in *E. angustifolia* with enthusiasm. Demand soon outstripped the supply coming from America, and, in an attempt to rapidly plant echinacea locally, the German firm Madeus and Company mistakenly purchased a quantity of *Echinacea purpurea* seeds. This historical accident is the reason why most echinacea today belongs to the *purpurea* species instead of *angustifolia*. Another family member, *Echinacea pallida*, is also used.

Echinacea was the number-one cold and flu remedy in the United States until it was displaced by sulfa antibiotics. Ironically, antibiotics are not effective for colds, while echinacea appears to offer some real help. Echinacea remains the primary remedy for minor respiratory infections in Germany, where over 1.3 million prescriptions are issued each year.

What Is Echinacea Used for Today?

Germany's Commission E authorizes the use of echinacea juice for "supportive treatment of recurrent infections of the upper respiratory tract and lower urinary tract" and echinacea root extracts for "supportive treatment of flu-like infections." Echinacea has become a wildly popular treatment for colds and flus in the United States as well, nearing the top of the charts for several years running.

The best scientific evidence about echinacea concerns its ability to help you recover from colds and minor flus more quickly. The old saying goes that a "cold lasts 7 days, but if you treat it, it will be over in a week." However, good evidence tells us that echinacea can actually help you get over colds much faster. It also appears to significantly reduce symptoms while you are sick.

Much weaker evidence suggests that echinacea may also be able to "abort" a cold, if taken at the first sign of symptoms, and perhaps slightly reduce the frequency of colds when taken regularly at the onset of cold season. (For more information on echinacea, see *The Natural Pharmacist Guide to Echinacea and Immunity*.)

What Is the Scientific Evidence for Echinacea?

Studies of echinacea have used all three species of the herb. We don't know which one is better, or whether they are all equivalent.

Reducing the Symptoms and Duration of Colds

Clinical studies with various species of echinacea have found benefits in lessening the symptoms and duration of colds. One double-blind study of 100 individuals with acute flu-like illnesses found that echinacea could significantly reduce cold symptoms.[1] Half of the group received a combination herb product containing *E. angustifolia*, the other half placebo. The participants rated the severity of symptoms of headache, lethargy, cough, and limb pain. In the treated group, symptoms were significantly less severe.

Another double-blind study of echinacea's effect on flu-like illnesses followed 180 people who were given either 450 mg or 900 mg of *E. purpurea* daily or placebo.[2] By about the third day, those participants receiving the higher dose of echinacea (900 mg) were doing significantly better than those in the placebo or low-dose echinacea groups.

Echinacea has also been found to reduce the time needed to get well. A double-blind placebo-controlled study using the *E. pallida* species followed 160 adults with recent onset of cold-like illnesses.[3] The results showed that treatment reduced the average period of illness from 13 days to about 9.5 days, compared to placebo. (These must have been bad colds to last so long!)

Finally, evidence from a double-blind study involving 120 people tells us that *E. purpurea* can cut in half the time it takes for your cold to "turn the corner" and start to get better. This study is described in the next section.

Preventing Colds

A double-blind study suggests that echinacea can not only make colds shorter and less severe, it can sometimes stop a cold that is just starting.[4] In this study, 120 people were given *E. purpurea* or a placebo as soon as they started showing signs of getting a cold.

Participants took either echinacea or placebo at a dosage of 20 drops every 2 hours for 1 day, then 20 drops three times a day for 9 more days. The results over the 10-day study period were promising. Fewer people in the echinacea group felt that their initial symptoms actually developed into "real" colds (40% of those taking echinacea versus 60% taking the placebo actually became ill). Also, among those who did come down with "real" colds, improvement in the symptoms started sooner in the echinacea group (4 days instead of 8 days). Both of these results were statistically significant. However, echinacea's ability to shorten the duration of colds was more dramatic.

A recent study attempted to discover whether the daily use of echinacea can prevent colds from even starting.[5] In this double-blind placebo-controlled trial, 302 healthy volunteers were given an alcohol tincture containing either *E. purpurea* root, *E. angustifolia* root, or placebo for 12 weeks. The results showed that *E. purpurea* was associated with perhaps a 20% decrease in the number of people who got sick, and *E. angustifolia* with a 10% decrease. However, the difference was not statistically significant. This means that the benefit, if any, was so small that it could have been due to chance alone.

In another double-blind placebo-controlled study, echinacea was found to offer some help, but only for those especially prone to colds.[6] The study involved 609 students at the University of Cologne. Half of the participants were treated with a German product containing *E. angustifolia* for at least 8 weeks; the other half received placebo.

In the group as a whole, echinacea did not significantly decrease the number of colds. However, of the 609 participants, 363 students were rated as particularly prone to infection, based on the number of colds each had developed the winter before. This relatively high-risk group did show a reduction in the number of colds they caught, compared to the control group: The infection-prone students developed on average 20% fewer colds (a statistically significant if not gigantic change).

This study suggests that for those who get sick easily, the regular use of echinacea may slightly decrease the incidence of winter colds. However, the bottom line is that echinacea is not very effective (if at all) as a long-term preventive treatment. It is better used directly at the onset of a cold to reduce its severity and duration or, with luck, to ward it off entirely.

Immune Stimulation

Both test-tube and animal studies have found that poly-saccharides found in echinacea can increase antibody production, raise white blood cell counts, and stimulate the activity of key white blood cells.[7–12] However, the meaningfulness of these studies has been questioned. Many other substances induce similar changes, including wheat, bamboo, rice, sugarcane, and chamomile, and none of these have ever been considered immune stimulants.[13] We don't know whether echinacea produces its effects by stimulating or strengthening the immune system, or in some altogether different way.

Dosage

Echinacea is usually taken at the first sign of a cold and continued for 7 to 14 days. The three species of echinacea are used interchangeably. The typical dosage of echinacea powdered extract is 300 mg 3 times a day. Alcohol tincture (1:5) is usually taken at a dosage of 3 to 4 ml 3 times daily, echinacea juice at a dosage of 2 to 3 ml 3 times daily, and whole dried root at 1 to 2 g 3 times daily.

There is no broad agreement on what ingredients should be standardized in echinacea tinctures and solid extracts. However, echinacea juice is often standardized to contain 2.4% of beta-1,2-fructofuranoside.

Many herbalists feel that liquid forms of echinacea are more effective than tablets or capsules, because they feel part of echinacea's benefit is due to activation of the tonsils through direct contact.[14]

Finally, goldenseal is frequently combined with echinacea in cold preparations. However, there is not a shred of evidence that oral goldenseal stimulates immunity, nor did traditional herbalists use it for this purpose.[15]

Safety Issues

Echinacea appears to be safe. Even when taken in very high doses, it has not been found to cause any toxic effects.[16,17] Reported side effects are also uncommon and usually limited to minor gastrointestinal symptoms, increased urination, and mild allergic reactions.[18] Studies dating back to the 1950s suggest that echinacea is safe in children.[19]

Germany's Commission E warns against using echinacea in cases of autoimmune disorders such as multiple sclerosis, lupus, and rheumatoid arthritis, as well as tuberculosis or leukocytosis. There are also rumors that echinacea should not be used by people with AIDS. These warnings are theoretical, based on fears that echinacea might actually activate immunity in the wrong way. But there is no evidence that echinacea use has actually harmed anyone with these diseases.

The Commission E monograph also recommends against using echinacea for more than 8 weeks. The safety of echinacea in young children, pregnant or nursing women, or those with severe liver or kidney disease has not been established. There are no known drug interactions.

ELDERBERRY
(SAMBUCUS NIGRA)

Principal Proposed Uses

Flus, colds

Other Proposed Uses

HIV, herpes

Native Americans used tea made from elderberry flowers to treat respiratory infections. They also used the leaves and flowers in poultices applied to wounds, and the bark, suitably aged, as a laxative. The berries are frequently made into beverages, pies, and preserves, but they have also been used to treat arthritis.

What Is Elderberry Used for Today?

Elderberry flowers are a potential rival for echinacea. Many clinicians feel that elderberry is actually more effective at shortening colds and flus than the latter, far more famous (and better-studied) herb. According to a preliminary double-blind study performed in Israel, a standardized elderberry extract reduced almost by half the recovery time from a particular strain of epidemic influenza.[1] Elderberry is being studied for potential activity against other viral illnesses as well, including HIV[2] and herpes.[3] Standardized elderberry extracts are seeing increasing use throughout Europe.

Dosage

Elderberry-flower tea is made by steeping 3 to 5 g of dried flowers in 1 cup of boiling water for 10 to 15 minutes. A typical dosage is 1 cup 3 times daily. Standardized extracts should be taken according to the directions on the product's label.

Safety Issues

Elderberry flowers are generally regarded as safe. Side effects are rare and consist primarily of occasional mild gastrointestinal distress or allergic reactions. Nonetheless, safety in young children, pregnant or nursing women, or those with severe liver or kidney disease is not established.

ELECAMPANE

(INULA HELENIUM)

Principal Proposed Uses

Chronic respiratory diseases, poor digestion

The Latin name of elecampane comes from Helen of Troy, who was supposed to have carried elecampane with her while being abducted from Sparta. Revered by the ancient Greeks and Romans, this herb was recommended for treating such diverse problems as indigestion, melancholy, sciatica, bronchitis, and asthma.

What Is Elecampane Used for Today?

Modern herbalists primarily regard elecampane as a long-term treatment for respiratory diseases such as asthma and bronchitis, especially when excessive mucus is a notable feature. Animal studies suggest that the oil of elecampane may help suppress coughs.[1] Unfortunately, no human trials of elecampane have been reported.

Elecampane is also sometimes recommended as a daily supplement to improve general digestion.

One of elecampane's constituents, alantolactone, has been used in concentrated form as a treatment for intestinal parasites,[2] but it isn't clear whether the whole herb is particularly effective for this purpose.

Dosage

A typical dosage of elecampane root is 1.5 to 4 g 3 times daily, either in capsule form or boiled in water as tea.

Safety Issues

The only reported adverse effects of elecampane are occasional allergic reactions. However, safety in young children, pregnant or nursing women, or those with severe liver or kidney disease is not established.

EPHEDRA a.k.a. MA HUANG
(EPHEDRA SINICA)

Principal Proposed Uses

Effective, but not recommended, for asthma and sinus congestion

Questionable Proposed Uses

Weight-loss aid, stimulant

The Chinese herb ma huang is a member of a primitive family of plants that look like thin, branching, connected straws. A related species, *Ephedra nevadensis*, grows wild in the American Southwest and is widely called "Mormon tea." However, only the Asian species of ephedra contains the active compounds ephedrine and pseudoephedrine.

Ma huang was traditionally used by Chinese herbalists during the early stages of respiratory infections, and also for the short-term treatment of certain kinds of asthma, eczema, hay fever, narcolepsy, and edema. However, ma huang was not supposed to be taken for an extended period of time, and people with less than robust constitutions were warned to use only low doses or avoid ma huang altogether. If these warnings had been heeded, perhaps some of the current problems with ephedra could have been avoided (see the discussion under What Is Ephedra Used for Today?).

Japanese chemists isolated ephedrine from ma huang at the turn of the century, and it soon became a primary treatment for asthma in the United States and abroad. Ephedra's other major ingredient, pseudoephedrine, became the decongestant Sudafed.

What Is Ephedra Used for Today?

Although it can still be found in a few over-the-counter asthma drugs, physicians seldom prescribe ephedrine anymore. The problem is that ephedrine mimics the effects of adrenaline and causes symptoms such as rapid heartbeat, high blood pressure, agitation, insomnia, nausea, and loss of appetite. The newer asthma drugs are much safer and easier to tolerate.

Recently, pills containing ephedrine have been sold as weight-loss aids and "natural" stimulants. Unfortunately, these products have been overused and combined with other stimulants, such as caffeine, resulting in severe overstimulation and even death in some people.[1] In 1997, the FDA proposed stiff limits on dietary supplements containing ephedrine, but they are presently under appeal by manufacturers who say they go too far. The FDA's intervention stemmed from unscrupulous manufacturers, who (mostly via the Internet) promoted ma huang as a natural hallucinogen ("herbal ecstasy"), and not as a bronchial decongestant. Dosages of ephedrine required to produce psychoactive effects are exceedingly toxic to the heart; the FDA has documented 38 deaths of otherwise healthy young people who reportedly used ephedrine for psychedelic purposes.

When used properly, ephedra may still be useful as a short-term treatment for sinus congestion and mild asthma, but I would not recommend it as conventional treatments are safer and cause fewer side effects.

Dosage

The dosage of ephedra should be adjusted according to the amount of the ephedrine it provides. A typical adult dosage is 12.5 to 25 mg of ephedrine 3 times daily. It should not be used for more than 1 week. In view of the documented dangers of ephedrine, medical supervision is highly recommended when using ephedra.

Safety Issues

Ephedra should *not* be taken by those with enlargement of the prostate, high blood pressure, heart disease, diabetes, hardening of the arteries, glaucoma, or hyperthyroidism.[2] Furthermore, never combine ephedra (or Sudafed) with monoamine-oxidase inhibitors (MAO inhibitors) such as Nardil, or fatal reactions may develop. If symptoms such as a rapid heart rate or a marked increase in blood pressure develop, reduce the dosage or simply stop taking it altogether.

Ephedra is not recommended for young children, pregnant or nursing women, or those with severe liver, heart or kidney disease.

EVENING PRIMROSE
(OENOTHERA BIENNIS)

Principal Proposed Uses

Fibrocystic breast disease (cyclic mastitis), diabetic neuropathy, general PMS symptoms, eczema

---

Evening primrose is a native American wildflower, named for the late-afternoon opening of its delicate flowers. Perhaps it should be described as a food supplement rather than an herb, for its oil has been popularized primarily as a source of gamma-linolenic acid (GLA), an essential fatty acid also found in black currant and borage.

Although many kinds of fat are unhealthy, essential fatty acids (EFAs) are as necessary as vitamins. There are two main kinds of EFAs: omega 3 and omega 6. The GLA in evening primrose is an omega-6 fatty acid.

The body ordinarily manufactures GLA from a common dietary fatty acid called linoleic acid. However, it appears that the body can't carry out this conversion properly under certain conditions, most notably diabetes, alcoholism, viral infections, high cholesterol, high fat intake, advanced age, infancy, and when deficiencies of pyridoxine (vitamin B_6), zinc, magnesium, biotin, or calcium are present.[1] Extra GLA may be very helpful in these situations.

What Is Evening Primrose Used for Today?

Many women experience cyclic episodes of breast tenderness often in association with PMS symptoms. This condition goes by various names, including *fibrocystic breast disease, cyclic mastalgia, cyclic mastitis,* and *mastodynia.* Evening primrose oil has become a medically accepted treatment for this condition in both the United States and Europe. Daily supplementation with evening primrose oil appears to produce substantial relief in perhaps 40 to 50% of women who try it.[2] However, this treatment takes 4 to 6 weeks for the first benefits to appear, and up to 4 to 8 months for full effect. Don't quit too soon!

Evening primrose oil is also said to be helpful for general PMS symptoms.

In Europe, evening primrose is also used to relieve symptoms of diabetic neuropathy. Additionally, it is a widely used and officially approved treatment for eczema in Great Britain, Ireland, Denmark, Germany, Spain, Greece, South Africa, Australia, and New Zealand.

For largely theoretical reasons, evening primrose oil has been suggested as a treatment for Raynaud's disease, Sjogren's disease, endometriosis, prostate disease, rheumatoid arthritis, chronic fatigue syndrome, and other conditions.

What Is the Scientific Evidence for Evening Primrose?

To date, there have been over 900 articles published on evening primrose oil or the GLA present in it.

Breast Tenderness

Investigation has found that women with this condition also have disturbances in levels of essential fatty acids.[3] Evening primrose oil may be able to correct this imbalance. In a small double-blind placebo-controlled study, the herbal treatment proved more effective than placebo.[4]

PMS

Although several studies have reported that evening primrose oil provides benefits in general PMS symptoms, they were all too badly flawed to prove anything.[5] (For more information on PMS, see *The Natural Pharmacist Guide to PMS.*)

Diabetic Neuropathy

Numerous studies in animals have found that evening primrose oil can protect nerves from diabetes-induced nerve injury.[6,7] More significantly, a double-blind study followed 111 patients from seven medical centers for a period of a year.[8] The results showed reduction in symptoms and signs of nerve injury. People with diabetes who had good blood sugar control improved the most. Earlier preliminary double-blind studies also found positive results.[9] (For more information on diabetes, see *The Natural Pharmacist Guide to Diabetes.*)

Eczema

The scientific evidence for evening primrose oil relieving eczema is modest and a bit contradictory. A recent double-blind study followed 58 children with eczema for 16 weeks.[10] Those treated with evening primrose oil did not show any significant benefit compared to the placebo group. However, a review of nine other preliminary double-blind studies (some of them unpublished) did find an overall positive effect, especially in relieving itching.[11]

Dosage

For cyclic breast pain, the standard dosage of evening primrose oil is 3 g daily. Children with eczema generally take 2 to 4 g daily, and people with diabetic neuropathy require 4 to 6 g daily. Evening primrose oil should be taken with food. Don't forget that full benefits may take over 6 months to develop.

For best results, you must also reduce your consumption of saturated and hydrogenated fats, such as those found in meat, butter, margarine, and some tropical vegetable oils.

Safety Issues

Animal studies suggest that evening primrose oil is completely nontoxic and noncarcinogenic.[12] Over 4,000 people have taken GLA or evening primrose oil in scientific studies, and no significant adverse effects have ever been noted. However, somewhat less than 2% of the study participants who took evening primrose oil complained of mild headaches and/or gastrointestinal distress, especially at higher dosages.[13,14]

Early case reports suggested the possibility that gamma-linolenic acid might worsen temporal lobe epilepsy or bipolar disorder, but there has been no later confirmation.[15,16]

The maximum safe dosage for young children, pregnant or nursing women, or those with severe liver or kidney disease has not been established.

EYEBRIGHT

(EUPHRASIA OFFICINALE L.)

Principal Proposed Uses

Eye infections

The herb eyebright has been used since the Middle Ages as an eyewash for infections and irritations. However, as much as one would like to believe that all traditions are wise, eyebright appears to have been selected for treating eye diseases not because it works particularly well, but because its petals look bloodshot.[1] This follows from the classic medieval philosophic attitude known as the *Doctrine of Signatures,* which states that herbs show their proper use by their appearance.

What Is Eyebright Used for Today?

Like many herbs, eyebright contains astringent substances and volatile oils that are probably at least slightly antibacterial. But there's no evidence that eyebright is particularly effective for treating eye diseases; Germany's Commission E recommends against using it. Warm compresses consisting of nothing but water (or ordinary black tea) are probably equally effective under the same conditions.

Eyebright tea is also sometimes taken internally to treat jaundice, respiratory infections, and memory loss. However, there is no evidence that it is effective for these conditions.

Dosage

Traditionally, eyebright tea is made by boiling 1 tablespoon of the herb in a cup of water. This is then used as an eyewash or taken internally up to 3 times daily.

Safety Issues

Eyebright can cause tearing of the eyes, itching, redness, and many other symptoms, probably due to direct irritation.[2] It appears to be safe when taken internally, but not many studies have been performed. Safety in young children, pregnant or nursing women, or those with severe liver or kidney disease is not established.

FENUGREEK

(TRIGONELLA FOENUMGRAECUM)

Principal Proposed Uses

Diabetes (blood sugar control, cholesterol levels)

For millennia, fenugreek has been used both as a medicine and as a food spice in Egypt, India, and the Middle East. It was traditionally recommended for the treatment of wounds, bronchitis, digestive problems, arthritis, kidney problems, and male reproductive conditions.

What Is Fenugreek Used for Today?

Present interest in fenugreek focuses on its benefits for those with diabetes or high cholesterol. Numerous animal studies and preliminary trials in humans have found that fenugreek can reduce blood sugar and serum cholesterol levels in people with diabetes.

What Is the Scientific Evidence for Fenugreek?

Small double-blind studies suggest that fenugreek can be helpful both for type 1 (childhood onset) and type 2 (adult onset) diabetes.

In one study of 60 people with type 2 diabetes, 25 mg a day of fenugreek led to significant improvements in overall blood sugar control, blood sugar elevations in response to a meal, and cholesterol levels.[1] Another study found benefits with only 15 mg of fenugreek daily.[2]

Finally, in a small double-blind, controlled study, people with type 1 diabetes were randomly prescribed either fenugreek at a dose of 50 gm twice daily as part of their lunch and dinner, or the same meals without the powder, each for 10 days. Those on the fenugreek diet had significant decreases in their fasting blood sugar.[3] (For more information on fenugreek in diabetes, see *The Natural Pharmacist Guide to Diabetes.*)

Dosage

Because the seeds of fenugreek are somewhat bitter, they are best taken in capsule form. The typical dosage is 5 to 30 g of defatted fenugreek taken 3 times a day with meals.

Safety Issues

As a commonly eaten food, fenugreek is generally regarded as safe. The only common side effect is mild gastrointestinal distress when it is taken in high doses.

Because fenugreek can lower blood sugar levels, it is advisable to seek medical supervision before combining it with diabetes medications.

Extracts made from fenugreek have been shown to stimulate uterine contractions in guinea pigs.[4] For this reason, pregnant women should not take fenugreek in dosages higher than is commonly used as a spice, perhaps 5 g daily. Besides concerns over pregnant women, safety in young children, nursing women, or those with severe liver or kidney disease has also not been established.

FEVERFEW

(TANACETUM PARTHENIUM)

Principal Proposed Uses

Migraine headaches (prevention and treatment)

Other Proposed Uses

Arthritis

Originally native to the Balkans, this relative of the common daisy was spread by deliberate planting throughout Europe and the Americas. Feverfew's feathery and aromatic leaves have long been used medicinally to improve childbirth, promote menstruation, induce abortions, relieve rheumatic pain, and treat severe headaches.

Contrary to popular belief, feverfew is not used for lowering fevers. Actually, "feverfew" is a corruption of the name "featherfoil."[1] Featherfoil became featherfew and ultimately feverfew. In a weird historical reversal, this name then led to a widespread belief among herbalists that feverfew could lower fevers. After a while they noticed that it didn't work, and then angrily rejected feverfew as a useless herb! Feverfew remained out of fashion until a serendipitous event occurred in the late 1970s.

At that time, the wife of the chief medical officer of the National Coal Board in England suffered from serious migraine headaches. When workers in the industry learned of this fact, a sympathetic miner suggested she try a folk treatment he had used. She followed his advice and chewed feverfew leaves. The results were dramatic: Her migraines disappeared almost completely.

Her husband was impressed, too. He used his high office to gain the ear of a physician who specialized in migraine headaches, Dr. E. Stewart Johnson of the

London Migraine Clinic. Johnson subsequently tried feverfew on 10 of his patients. The results were so good that he subsequently gave the herb to 270 of his patients. A whopping 70% reported considerable relief.

Thoroughly excited now, Dr. Johnson enrolled 17 feverfew-using patients in an interesting type of double-blind study: Half continued to use feverfew, and the other half were transferred, without their knowledge, to a placebo.[2] Over a period of 6 months, the patients with drawn from feverfew demonstrated a dramatic increase in headaches, nausea, and vomiting.

Unfortunately, this study didn't prove much. It was too small and, because the patients were already feverfew users, it didn't say anything about the effectiveness of feverfew in the population at large. (Presumably, the participants used feverfew because they already knew that the herb worked for them.) Nonetheless, the study brought a flood of response from the public, and ultimately led to the properly performed double-blind experiments described below.

For many years, it was assumed that the active ingredient in feverfew was a substance named parthenolide. Numerous articles were published explaining exactly how parthenolide prevented migraines, stating that it caused platelets to release serotonin and reduce the synthesis of prostaglandins, leukotrienes, and thromboxanes.[3–6] Based on this premature explanation, indignant authors complained that samples of feverfew on the market varied as much as 10 to 1 in their parthenolide content. No less an authority than herbal expert Varro Tyler said, "Standardization of the herbal material on the basis of its parthenolide content is urgently required if this potentially valuable herb is to be used effectively." [7]

However, everyone was jumping the gun. A recent study found that an extract of feverfew standardized to a high-parthenolide content is entirely ineffective.[8] Apparently, this high-parthenolide extract lacked some essential substance or group of substances present in the whole leaf. What those substances may be, however, remains mysterious.

What Is Feverfew Used for Today?

Feverfew is primarily used for prevention of chronic, recurrent migraine headaches. It must be taken religiously every day for best results. (For more information on migraines, see *The Natural Pharmacist Guide to Feverfew and Migraines*.)

Feverfew is also sometimes used at the onset of a migraine attack. It is not believed to be effective for cluster or tension headaches.

It is important to remember that serious diseases may occasionally first present themselves as migraine-type headaches. For this reason, proper medical diagnosis is essential if you suddenly start having migraines without a previous history, or if the pattern of your migraines changes significantly.

Feverfew is sometimes recommended as a treatment for arthritis, but there is no evidence that it works.

What Is the Scientific Evidence for Feverfew?

Three double-blind studies have been performed to evaluate feverfew's effectiveness as a preventive treatment for migraines. Two returned positive results, the other negative.

The Nottingham trial followed 59 individuals for 8 months.[9] For 4 months, half received a daily capsule of powdered feverfew leaf; the other half took placebo. The groups were then switched and followed for an additional 4 months. Treatment with feverfew produced a 24% reduction in the number of migraines and a significant decrease in nausea and vomiting during the headaches.

A recent Israeli study of 57 people with migraines found a significant decrease in severity of migraine headaches.[10] Unfortunately, it did not report whether there was any change in the frequency of migraines. This study also used powdered feverfew leaf.

However, a Dutch study involving 50 people showed no difference whatsoever between placebo and a special feverfew extract standardized to parthenolide content.[11] As mentioned above, the explanation appears to be that parthenolide is not the active ingredient in feverfew.

Dosage

Given the recent confusion surrounding parthenolide, previous dosage recommendations for feverfew based on parthenolide content have been cast in doubt. At the present time, the best recommendation is probably to take 80 to 100 mg of powdered whole feverfew leaf daily.

When taken at the onset of a migraine headache, higher amounts of feverfew are often used. However, the optimum dosage has not been determined.

Safety Issues

Among the many thousands of people who use feverfew as a folk medicine in England, there have been no reports of serious toxicity. Animal studies suggest that feverfew is essentially nontoxic.[12]

In the 8-month Nottingham trial, there were no significant differences in side effects between the treated and control groups.[13] There were also no changes in measurements on blood tests and urinalysis.

In a survey involving 300 people, 11.3% reported mouth sores from chewing feverfew leaf, occasionally accompanied by general inflammation of tissues in the mouth.[14] A smaller percentage reported mild gastrointestinal distress.[15]

However, mouth sores do not seem to occur in people who use encapsulated feverfew leaf powder, the usual form.

In view of its use as a folk remedy to promote abortions, feverfew should probably not be taken during pregnancy.

Safety in young children, pregnant or nursing women, or those with severe kidney or liver disease has not been established.

GARLIC
(ALLIUM SATIVUM)

Principal Proposed Uses

Atherosclerosis (lowering cholesterol, reducing blood pressure, "thinning" the blood), heart attack prevention

Other Proposed Uses

Cancer prevention, topical antibiotic and antifungal, immune stimulant

Probably Ineffective Uses

Oral antibiotic, ear infections

The story of garlic's role in human history could fill a book, as indeed it has, many times. Its species name, *sativum*, means cultivated, indicating that garlic does not grow in the wild. So fond have humans been of this herb that garlic can be found almost everywhere in the world, from Polynesia to Siberia. Interestingly, as far back as the first century A.D., Dioscorides wrote of garlic's ability to "clear the arteries."

From Roman antiquity through World War I, garlic poultices were used to prevent wound infections. The famous microbiologist, Louis Pasteur, performed some of the original work showing that garlic could kill bacteria. In 1916, the British government issued a general plea for the public to supply it with garlic in order to meet wartime needs. Garlic was called "Russian penicillin" during World War II because, after running out of antibiotics, the Russian government turned to this ancient treatment for its soldiers.

Conventional doctors in the United States continued to use garlic even when they had abandoned nearly all other herbs. After World War II, Sandoz Pharmaceuticals manufactured a garlic compound for intestinal spasms, and the Van Patten Company produced another for lowering blood pressure.

In the 1950s, garlic finally fell completely out of favor with American physicians. European physicians, continued to investigate garlic.

What Is Garlic Used for Today?

In Europe, garlic has come to be seen as an all-around treatment for preventing atherosclerosis, the cause of heart disease and strokes. As we'll see in the following discussion, moderately good studies have found that certain forms of garlic can lower total cholesterol levels by about 9 to 12%, as well as possibly improve the ratio of good and bad cholesterol. Garlic also appears to reduce blood pressure (although only modestly), protect against free radicals and slow blood coagulation. Putting all these benefits together, garlic may be a broad-spectrum treatment for arterial disease.

Preliminary evidence suggests that regular use of garlic may help prevent cancer. While eating garlic is commonly stated to raise immunity, there is no real evidence that this is the case. Garlic is an effective antibiotic when it contacts the tissue directly, but there is no reason to believe that it will work in this way if you take it by mouth.

Finally, garlic oil products are often recommended for children's ear infections. While these products may reduce pain, it is very unlikely that they have any actual effect on the infection because the eardrum is in the way. (For more information on garlic, see *The Natural Pharmacist Guide to Garlic and Cholesterol.*)

What Is the Scientific Evidence for Garlic?

The science behind using garlic to prevent atherosclerosis is moderately strong, although there are some contradictions in the research record.

Garlic preparations have been found to slow hardening of the arteries in animals, reducing the size of plaque deposits by nearly 50%.[1,2] Garlic appears to function somewhat like prescription drugs by interfering with the manufacture of cholesterol.[3,4,5]

Garlic extracts have been found to reduce blood pressure in dogs and rats,[6] and numerous animal studies suggest that it can reduce blood clotting and neutralize free radicals.[7–13]

High Cholesterol

At least 28 controlled clinical studies of using garlic to treat elevated cholesterol were published between 1985 and 1995. Together, they suggest that garlic can lower cholesterol by about 9 to 12%.[14,15] Virtually all of these studies used garlic standardized to alliin content (see the discussion under Dosage). Garlic oil does not seem to be effective.

One of the best of these studies was conducted in Germany and published in 1990.[16] A total of 261 patients at 30 medical centers were given either 800 mg of standardized garlic daily or placebo. Over the course of 16 weeks, patients in the treated group experienced a 12% drop in total cholesterol and a 17% decrease in triglyceride levels. The greatest benefits occurred in patients with initial cholesterol levels of 250 to 300 mg/dL.

Another double-blind study, reported in 1996, followed 41 men with cholesterol readings of 220 to 290 mg/dL.[17] The men received either placebo or 7.2 g of aged garlic extract daily for 6 months; then their treatments were switched for 4 months. The results showed a 7% decrease in total serum cholesterol and a 4% decrease in LDL cholesterol in the garlic-treated group. There was also a 5.5% decrease in blood pressure.

One widely quoted study compared garlic to the standard cholesterol-lowering drug bezafibrate.[18] Although the results showed them to be equally effective, the study was not designed properly, so the results mean little. Both groups in the study improved their diets dramatically, which could have easily overshadowed real differences between the treatments.

In contrast to these positive results, a couple of other studies have shown no benefit with garlic powder. One study, published in 1996, followed 115 individuals with total cholesterol concentrations of 231 to 328 mg/dL, half of whom received 900 mg daily of a standard garlic extract standardized to contain 1.3% allicin.[19] The results showed no significant difference between the treated and placebo groups. Another negative study was reported in 1995.[20]

These discrepancies are troubling, but they occur in the research record of standard drugs as well. Overall, the evidence for garlic powder is strongly favorable.

It can be said with some certainty that garlic oil is not effective for lowering cholesterol.[21]

High Blood Pressure

Numerous studies have found that garlic lowers blood pressure slightly, usually in the neighborhood of 5 to 10% more than placebo.[22,23] However, all of these studies suffered from significant flaws, and most were performed on people without high blood pressure.

One of the best studies followed 47 subjects with an average starting blood pressure of 171/101.[24] Over a period of 12 weeks, half were treated with 600 mg of garlic powder daily standardized to 1.3% alliin, the other half were given placebo. The results showed a statistically significant drop of 11% in the systolic blood pressure and 13% in the diastolic pressure. (Blood pressure also fell in the placebo group, by 5% and 4% respectively, so the actual improvement due to garlic is somewhat less than it first appears.) Some garlic studies have been criticized on the basis of the participants being able to tell whether they were being given real garlic or placebo by detecting the garlic odor, but the study authors state that regular questioning of the participants revealed that they could not tell which group they were in.

Another study suggests that garlic's effects increase if it is given a longer time to act. In a 16-week open trial, about 40 subjects with mild hypertension (average blood pressure of 151/96) were given either 600 mg 3 times daily of a garlic preparation standardized to 1.3% alliin (an unusually high dose).[25] The group treated with standardized garlic started with an average blood pressure of 151/96. At 4 weeks, there was a 10% drop in systolic blood pressure, and at 16 weeks the improvement reached 19%. Similar progressive changes occurred in the diastolic blood pressure.

Direct Effects on Hardening of the Arteries
A recent observational study of 200 individuals suggests that garlic can affect hardening of the arteries by some unidentified means other than lowering cholesterol or blood pressure.[26] The study measured the flexibility of the aorta, the main artery exiting the heart.

Preventing Heart Attacks
In one study, 432 individuals who had suffered a heart attack were given either garlic juice in milk daily (yum!) or

no treatment at all over a period of 3 years.[27] The results showed a significant reduction of second heart attacks and about a 50% reduction in death rate among those taking garlic.

Cancer Prevention

Several large studies strongly suggest that a diet high in garlic can prevent cancer. In one of the best, the Iowa Women's Study, a group of 41,837 women were questioned as to their lifestyle habits in 1986, and then followed continuously in subsequent years. At the 4-year follow-up, questionnaires showed that women whose diets included significant quantities of garlic were approximately 30% less likely to develop colon cancer.[28]

The interpretations of studies like this one are always a bit controversial. For example, it's possible that the women who ate a lot of garlic also made other healthy lifestyle choices. While researchers looked at this possibility very carefully and concluded that garlic was a common factor, it is not clear that they are right. What is really needed to settle the question is an intervention trial, where some people are given garlic and others are given a placebo. However, none has yet been performed.[29]

Antimicrobial

There is no question that raw garlic can kill a wide variety of microorganisms by direct contact, including fungi, bacteria, viruses, and protozoa.[30] This may explain why applying garlic directly to a wound was traditionally done to prevent infection. But there is no evidence that taking garlic orally can kill organisms throughout the body.[31–35] Thus, it's not an antiobiotic in the usual sense. It's more like Bacitracin ointment. However, garlic can cause burns when it is applied to the skin (see Dosage).

Dosage

A great deal of controversy exists over the proper dosage and form of garlic. Most everyone agrees that one or two raw garlic cloves a day are adequate, but virtual trade wars have taken place over the potency and effectiveness of various dried, aged, or deodorized garlic preparations. The problem has to do with the way garlic is naturally constructed.

A relatively odorless substance, alliin, is one of the most important compounds in garlic. When garlic is crushed or cut, an enzyme called allinase is brought in contact with alliin, turning it into allicin. The allicin itself then rapidly breaks down into entirely different compounds. Allicin is most responsible for garlic's strong odor. It can also blister the skin and kill bacteria, viruses, and fungi. Presumably the garlic plant uses allicin as a form of protection from pests and parasites. It also may provide much of the medicinal benefits of garlic.

When you powder garlic to put it in a capsule, it acts like cutting the bulb. The chain reaction starts: Alliin contacts allinase, yielding allicin, which then breaks down. Unless something is done to prevent this process, garlic powder won't have any alliin or allicin left by the time you buy it.

Some garlic producers declare that alliin and allicin have nothing to do with garlic's effectiveness and simply sell products without it. This is particularly true of aged powdered garlic and garlic oil. But others feel certain that allicin is absolutely essential. However, in order to make garlic relatively odorless, they must prevent the alliin from turning into allicin until the product is consumed. To accomplish this feat, they engage in marvelously complex manufacturing processes, each unique and proprietary. How well each of these methods work is a matter of finger-pointing controversy.

The best that can be said at this point is that in most of the studies that found cholesterol-lowering powers in garlic, the daily dosage supplied at least 10 mg of alliin. This is sometimes stated in terms of how much allicin will be created from that alliin. The number you should look for is 4 to 5 mg of "allicin potential."

Alliin-free aged garlic also appears to be effective when taken at a dose of 1 to 7.2 g daily. (For more information on this controversial topic, see *The Natural Pharmicist Guide to Garlic and Cholesterol.*)

Safety Issues

As a commonly used food, garlic is on the FDA's "generally regarded as safe" (GRAS) list. Rats have been fed gigantic doses of aged garlic (2,000 mg per kilogram body weight) for 6 months without any signs of negative effects.[36] Unfortunately, there do not appear to be any animal toxicity studies on the most commonly used form of garlic—powdered garlic standardized to alliin content.

The only common side effect of garlic is unpleasant breath odor. Even "odorless garlic" produces an offensive smell in up to 50% of those who use it.[37]

Other side effects occur only rarely. For example, a study that followed 1,997 people who were given a normal dose of deodorized garlic daily over a 16-week period showed a 6% incidence of nausea, a 1.3% incidence of dizziness on standing (perhaps a sign of low blood pressure), and a 1.1% incidence of allergic reactions.[38] These are very low percentages in comparison to those usually reported in drug studies. There were also a few reports of bloating, headaches, sweating, and dizziness.

When raw garlic is taken in excessive doses, it can cause numerous symptoms, such as stomach upset, heartburn, nausea, vomiting, diarrhea, flatulence, facial flushing, rapid pulse, and insomnia.

Topical garlic can cause skin irritation, blistering, and even third-degree burns, so be very careful about applying garlic directly to the skin.

Since garlic "thins" the blood, it is not a good idea to take high-potency garlic pills immediately prior to surgery or labor and delivery, due to the risk of excessive bleeding. Similarly, garlic should not be combined with blood-thinning drugs, such as aspirin or Trental (pentoxifylline). Finally, garlic could conceivably interact with natural products with blood-thinning properties, such as ginkgo or high-dose vitamin E.

Garlic is presumed to be safe for pregnant women (except just before delivery) and nursing mothers, although this has not been proven.

GENTIAN

(GENTIANA LUTEA)

Principal Proposed Uses

Poor appetite, poor digestion

For reasons that aren't entirely clear, bitter plants have the capacity to stimulate appetite, and gentian ranks high on the scale of bitterness. Two of its constituents, gentiopicrin and amarogentin, taste bitter even when diluted by a factor of 50,000![1]

In traditional European herbology, gentian and other bitter herbs are believed to strengthen the digestive system when taken over a period of time. However, in Chinese medicine, gentian is regarded as a rather intense herb that should seldom be taken over the long term. I'm not sure which view is right, although I tend to lean toward the Chinese viewpoint, and only recommend gentian for short-term use.

What Is Gentian Used for Today?

Gentian extracts are widely sold in liquor stores under the name "bitters," for the purpose of increasing appetite. Tinctures are also sold medicinally for the same purpose.

Dosage

A typical dosage of gentian is 20 drops of tincture 15 minutes before meals. To make the intensely bitter taste more tolerable, you can mix the tincture in juice or water.

Safety Issues

Gentian is somewhat mutagenic, meaning that it can cause changes in the DNA of bacteria.[2] For this reason, gentian should not be taken during pregnancy. Safety in young children, nursing women, or those with severe liver or kidney disease is also not established.

In the short term, gentian rarely causes any side effects, except for occasional worsening of ulcer pain and heartburn. (For some people, it relieves stomach problems.)

GINGER

(ZINGIBER OFFICINALE)

Principal Proposed Uses

Nausea (e.g., motion sickness, morning sickness in pregnancy, post-surgical nausea)

Native to southern Asia, ginger is a 2- to 4-foot perennial that produces grass-like leaves up to a foot long and almost an inch wide. Ginger root, as it is called in the grocery store, actually consists of the underground stem of the plant, with its bark-like outer covering scraped off.

Ginger has been used as food and medicine for millennia. Arabian traders carried ginger root from China and India to be used as a food spice in ancient Greece and Rome, and tax records from the second century A.D. show that ginger was a delightful source of revenue to the Roman treasury. Presently, the annual production of ginger exceeds 2 million pounds.

Chinese medical texts from the fourth century B.C. suggest that ginger is effective in treating nausea, diarrhea, stomachaches, cholera, toothaches, bleeding, and rheumatism. Ginger was later used by Chinese herbalists to treat a variety of respiratory conditions, including coughs and the early stages of colds.

Ginger's modern use dates back to the early 1980s, when a scientist named D. Mowrey noticed that ginger-filled capsules reduced his nausea during an episode of flu. Inspired by this, he performed the first double-blind study of ginger. Germany's Commission E subsequently approved ginger as a treatment for indigestion and motion sickness.

One of the most prevalent ingredients in fresh ginger is the pungent substance gingerol. However, when ginger is dried and stored, its gingerol rapidly converts to the substances shogaol and zingerone. Which, if any, of these substances is most important has not been determined.

What Is Ginger Used for Today?

Ginger has become widely accepted as a treatment for nausea. Even some conventional medical texts suggest ginger for the treatment of the nausea and vomiting of pregnancy, although others are more cautious.

Ginger is also used for motion sickness. Medications, such as meclizine, are usually more effective, but they can cause drowsiness. Some conventional physicians recommend ginger over other motion-sickness drugs for older people who are unusually sensitive to drowsiness or loss of balance.

European physicians sometimes give their patients ginger before and just after surgery to prevent the nausea that many people experience on awakening from anesthesia. However, this treatment should only be attempted with a doctor's approval.

Ginger has been suggested as a treatment for numerous other conditions, including migraine headaches, rheumatoid arthritis, high cholesterol, burns, ulcers, depression, impotence, and liver toxicity. However, there is negligible evidence for these uses.

In traditional Chinese medicine, hot ginger tea taken at the first sign of a cold is believed to offer the possibility of averting the infection. However, once more there is no scientific evidence for this use.

What Is the Scientific Evidence for Ginger?

The evidence for ginger's effectiveness is mixed. It has been suggested that, in some negative studies, poor-quality ginger powder might have been used.[1] In general, while most antinausea drugs influence the brain and the inner ear, ginger appears to act only on the stomach.[2]

Motion Sickness

The first ginger study followed 36 college students with a known tendency toward motion sickness.[3] They were treated with either ginger or the standard nausea drug dimenhydrinate, and then placed in a rotating chair to see how much they could stand. Both treatments seemed about equally effective.

Another study also found equivalent benefit between ginger and dimenhydrinate in a group of 60 passengers on a cruise through rough seas.[4] A later study of 79 Swedish naval cadets found that ginger could decrease vomiting and cold sweating, but didn't significantly decrease nausea and vertigo.[5]

However, a 1984 study funded by NASA found that ginger was not any more effective than placebo.[6] Two other small studies have also failed to find any benefit.[7,8] The reason for the discrepancy may lie in the type of ginger used, or the severity of the stimulant used to bring on motion sickness.

Nausea and Vomiting of Pregnancy

A preliminary double-blind study performed in Denmark concluded that ginger can significantly reduce the nausea and vomiting often associated with pregnancy. Effects became apparent in 19 of 27 women after 4 days of treatment, although the relief was far from total.[9]

Post-Surgical Nausea

A double-blind British study compared the effects of ginger, placebo, and metoclopramide in the treatment of nausea following gynecological surgery.[10] The results in 60 women indicated that both treatments produced similar benefits as compared to placebo.

A similar British study followed 120 women receiving elective laparoscopic gynecological surgery.[11] Whereas nausea and vomiting developed in 41% of the participants given placebo, in the groups treated with ginger or metoclopramide (Reglan) these symptoms developed in only 21% and 27% respectively.

However, a double-blind study of 108 people undergoing similar surgery found no benefit with ginger as compared to placebo.[12] Actually, ginger in doses of 0.5 and 1 g worsened nausea symptoms. Negative results were also seen in another recent study of 120 women.[13]

Dosage

For most purposes, the standard dosage of powdered ginger is 1 to 4 g daily taken in 2 to 4 divided doses.

To prevent motion sickness, it is probably best to begin treatment 1 or 2 days before the trip and continue it throughout the period of travel.

In the nausea and vomiting of pregnancy, the best form of ginger is probably freshly brewed tea, made from boiled ginger root and diluted to taste. If chilled, carbonated, and sweetened, this would become the original form of ginger ale, a famous antinausea beverage. Powdered ginger can be used as well.

Safety Issues

Ginger is on the FDA's GRAS (generally recognized as safe) list as a food, and the treatment dosages of ginger are comparable to dietary usages.

Like onions and garlic, extracts of ginger inhibit blood coagulation in test-tube experiments.[14,15,16] This has led to a theoretical concern that ginger should not be combined with drugs such as Coumadin (warfarin), heparin, or even aspirin. However, European studies with actual oral ginger in normal quantities have not found any significant effect on blood coagulation.[17,18,19]

No side effects have been observed with ginger at recommended dosages.

GINKGO
(GINKGO BILOBA)

Principal Proposed Uses

Memory and mental function (e.g., Alzheimer's disease, non-Alzheimer's dementia, ordinary age-related memory loss)

Other Proposed Uses

Impaired circulation in the legs (intermittent claudication), fluid retention related to the menstrual cycle, macular degeneration, impotence, tinnitus

Traceable back 300 million years, the ginkgo is the oldest surviving species of tree. Although it died out in Europe during the Ice Age, ginkgo survived in China, Japan, and other parts of East Asia. It has been cultivated extensively for both ceremonial and medical purposes, and some particularly revered trees have been lovingly tended for over 1,000 years.

In traditional Chinese herbology, tea made from ginkgo seeds has been used for numerous problems, most particularly asthma and other respiratory illnesses. The leaf was not used. But in the 1950s, German researchers started to investigate the medical possibilities of ginkgo leaf extracts rather than remedies using the seeds. Thus, modern ginkgo preparations are not the same as the traditional Chinese herb, and the comparisons often drawn are incorrect.

What Is Ginkgo Used for Today?

Presently, ginkgo is the most widely prescribed herb in Germany, reaching a total prescription count of over 6 million in 1995.[1] German physicians consider it to be as effective as any drug treatment for Alzheimer's disease and other severe forms of memory and mental function decline.

We do not know for sure whether ginkgo is helpful in ordinary, age-related memory loss, although there are logical reasons to believe it might be. (See *The Natural Pharmacist Guide to Ginkgo and Memory* for more information.)

Germany's Commission E also recommends ginkgo for the treatment of restricted circulation in the legs due to hardening of the arteries (intermittent claudication). Recently, ginkgo has attracted interest for possibly reversing the impotence caused by certain antidepressant drugs.

One study suggests that ginkgo may be helpful to relieve the bloating and fluid retention of PMS.[2] (See *The Natural Pharmacist Guide to PMS* for more information on PMS treatments.)

Additionally, ginkgo is used to treat ringing in the ears (tinnitus) and macular degeneration, although there is little evidence that it is effective for these purposes.

What Is the Scientific Evidence for Ginkgo?

The scientific record for gingko is extensive and impressive. Studies have found that ginkgo extracts can improve circulation.[3,4] We don't know exactly how ginkgo does this, but unknown constituents in the herb appear to make the blood more fluid, reduce the tendency toward blood clots, extend the life of a natural blood vessel–relaxing substance, and act as an antioxidant.[5,6] However, ginkgo's influence on mental function probably has nothing to do with its effects on circulation.

Impaired Mental Function in the Elderly

In the past, European physicians believed that the cause of mental deterioration with age (senile dementia) was reduced circulation in the brain. Since ginkgo can improve circulation, they assumed that ginkgo was simply getting more blood to brain cells and thereby making them work better. However, the modern understanding of age-related memory loss and mental impairment no longer considers chronically restricted circulation a primary issue. Ginkgo (and other drugs used for dementia) most likely function by directly stimulating nerve-cell activity and protecting nerve cells from further injury.[7]

According to a 1992 article published in *Lancet,* over 40 double-blind controlled trials have evaluated the benefits of ginkgo in treating age-related mental decline.[8] Of these, 8 were rated of good quality, involving a total of about 1,000 people and producing positive results in all but one study. The authors of the *Lancet* article felt that the evidence was strong enough to conclude that ginkgo extract is an effective treatment for this condition.

Studies since 1992 have verified this conclusion, both in people with Alzheimer's disease and those without the disorder.[9,10] Interestingly, European physicians are so certain that ginkgo is effective that it's become hard for them to perform scientific studies of the herb. To them, it's unethical to give Alzheimer's patients a placebo when they could take ginkgo instead and have additional months of useful life.[11]

This objection doesn't apply in the United States, where physicians generally do not believe that ginkgo is effective. A recent study published in the *Journal of the American Medical Association* reported on the results of a year-long double-blind trial of *Ginkgo biloba* in over 300 individuals with Alzheimer's disease or other forms of severe age-related mental decline.[12] Participants were given either 40 mg of the ginkgo extract or placebo 3 times daily. The results showed significant (but not miraculous) improvements in the treated group.

Contrary to some reports, the type of ginkgo used in the study is identical to standardized extracts widely available in the United States.

Impaired Circulation in the Legs (Intermittent Claudication)

In intermittent claudication, impaired circulation can cause a severe, cramp-like pain in one's legs after walking only a short distance. According to Germany's Commission E, at least four reasonably good double-blind studies have found that ginkgo can increase pain-free walking distance by 75 to 500 feet. [13]

One double-blind study enrolled 111 people for 24 weeks.[14] Subjects were measured for pain-free walking distance by walking up a 12% slope on a treadmill at 3 kilometers per hour (about 2 miles per hour). At the beginning of treatment, both the placebo and ginkgo groups were able to walk about 350 feet without pain. By the end of the trial, both groups had improved significantly (the power of placebo is amazing!). However, the ginkgo group improved more: Participants taking ginkgo achieved an average of 500 feet while those in the placebo group reached only 415 feet, an improvement of 85 feet for the ginkgo group. This was not miraculous, but it was still significant.

Positive results were also seen in another recent, double-blind placebo-controlled study. [15]

Fluid Retention Related to the Menstrual Cycle

One double-blind placebo-controlled study evaluated the benefits of *Ginkgo biloba* extract in women who experience fluid retention related to the menstrual cycle.[16] A group of 165 women, treated with either 80 mg of ginkgo extract twice daily or a placebo, were followed for one menstrual cycle. The results showed that ginkgo can significantly reduce some symptoms of PMS, especially bloating and breast swelling.

Macular Degeneration

One preliminary double-blind study suggests that ginkgo may improve macular degeneration.[17]

Impotence

Although there is no double-blind evidence at the time of this writing, case reports suggest that ginkgo can reverse the impotence caused by drugs in the Prozac family.[18]

Dosage

The standard dosage of ginkgo is 40 to 80 mg 3 times daily of a 50:1 extract standardized to contain 24% ginkgo-flavone glycosides.

Safety Issues

Ginkgo appears to be safe. Extremely high doses have been given in animals for long periods of time without serious consequences.[19] Safety in young children, pregnant or nursing women, or those with severe liver or kidney disease, however, has not been established.

In all the clinical trials of ginkgo up through 1991 combined, involving a total of almost 10,000 participants, the incidence of side effects produced by ginkgo extract was extremely small. There were 21 cases of gastrointestinal discomfort, and even fewer cases of headaches, dizziness, and allergic skin reactions.[20]

Contact with live ginkgo plants can cause severe allergic reactions, and ingestion of ginkgo seeds can be dangerous.

German medical authorities do not believe that ginkgo possesses any serious drug interactions.[21] However, because of ginkgo's "blood-thinning" effects, some experts warn that it should not be combined with blood-thinning drugs such as Coumadin (warfarin), heparin, aspirin, and Trental (pentoxifylline), and use of such drugs was prohibited in most of the double-blind trials of ginkgo. It is also possible that ginkgo could cause bleeding problems if combined with natural blood thinners, such as garlic and high-dose vitamin E. There have been two case reports in highly regarded journals of subdural hematoma (bleeding in the skull) and hyphema (spontaneous bleeding into the iris chamber) in association with ginkgo use. [22,23]

GINSENG

(PANAX GINSENG, PANAX QUINQUEFOLIUS)

Principal Proposed Uses

Adaptogen (improving resistance to stress), strengthening immunity, enhancing mental function, improving blood sugar control in people with diabetes

Other Proposed Uses

Increasing exercise capacity

There are actually three different herbs commonly called ginseng: Asian ginseng *(Panax ginseng)*, American ginseng *(Panax quinquefolius)* and Siberian "ginseng" *(Eleutherococcus senticosus)*. The latter herb is actually not ginseng at all, but the Russian scientists responsible for promoting it believe that it functions identically.

Asian ginseng is a perennial herb with a taproot resembling the human body. It grows in northern China, Korea, and Russia; its close relative, *Panax quinquefolius*, is cultivated in the United States. Because ginseng must be grown for 5 years before it is harvested, it commands a high price, with top-quality roots easily selling for more than $10,000. Dried, unprocessed ginseng root is called "white ginseng," and steamed, heat-dried root is "red ginseng." Chinese herbalists believe that each form has its own particular benefits.

Ginseng is widely regarded by the public as a stimulant, but according to everyone who uses it seriously that isn't the right description. In traditional Chinese herbology, *Panax ginseng* was used to strengthen the digestion and the lungs, calm the spirit, and increase overall energy. When the Russian scientist Israel I. Brekhman became interested in the herb prior to World War II, he came up with a new idea about ginseng. He decided that it was an adaptogen.

The term *adaptogen* refers to a hypothetical treatment described as follows: An adaptogen should help the body adapt to stresses of various kinds, whether heat, cold, exertion, trauma, sleep deprivation, toxic exposure, radiation, infection, or psychological stress. Furthermore, an adaptogen should cause no side effects, be effective in treating a wide variety of illnesses, and help return an organism toward balance no matter what may have gone wrong.

Perhaps the only indisputable example of an adaptogen is healthy lifestyle. By eating right, exercising regularly, and generally living a life of balance and moderation, you will increase your physical fitness and ability to resist illnesses of all types. Whether there are any substances that can do as much remains unclear. However, Brekhman felt certain that ginseng produced similarly universal benefits.

Interestingly, traditional Chinese medicine (where ginseng comes from) does not entirely agree. There is no one-size-fits-all in Chinese medical theory. Like any other herb, ginseng is said to be helpful for those people who need its particular effects, and neutral or harmful for others. But in Europe, Brekhman's concept has taken hold, and ginseng is widely believed to be a universal adaptogen.

In the 1940s, Brekhman decided that a much less expensive herb, *Eleutherococcus senticosus*, is just as good as ginseng. A thorny bush that grows much more rapidly than true ginseng, this later received the misleading name of "Siberian" or "Russian ginseng." Contrary to some reports, its chemical makeup is completely unrelated to that of *Panax ginseng*.

What Is Ginseng Used for Today?

If Brekhman is right, ginseng (whether *Eleutherococcus* or *Panax*) should be the right treatment for most of us. Modern life is tremendously stressful, and if an herb could help us withstand it, it would be a terrifically useful herb indeed. Ginseng is widely used for this purpose in Russia and Eastern Europe. However, the scientific basis for this use is not strong. There have been a few good studies of ginseng for certain more specific purposes: strengthening immunity, stimulating the mind, helping to control diabetes, and improving physical performance capacity (sports performance).

What Is the Scientific Evidence for Ginseng?

There have been thousands of research papers published on ginseng. Unfortunately, nearly all involved animals who received injections of ginseng extracts directly into the abdomen. There are only a few good double-blind human studies of ginseng taken by mouth.

Animal Studies

In animals, ginseng injections have been found to increase stamina; improve mental function; protect against radiation, infections, toxins, exhaustion, and stress; and activate white blood cells.[1] If you put these studies together, injected ginseng truly does appear to be an adaptogen, as advertised.

However, having ginseng injected into the abdomen is strikingly different from taking it by mouth. It not only enters the body directly without going through the digestive tract, but for all we know, an injection into the abdomen may itself stimulate numerous bodily changes.

Open Studies

Although many scientific trials of ginseng involve people, some with enormous numbers of participants, most were not double-blind. This makes the results nearly meaningless.

For example, one widely quoted study followed over 50,000 employees at a Soviet automobile plant who were given *Eleutherococcus* daily during November and December. Plant records showed that the frequency of respiratory infections fell by 40%.[2] However, without a control group, it isn't clear how many infections would have been expected without any treatment. Perhaps it was a milder winter, for example. Furthermore, since the participants knew they were being treated, the placebo effect was given full reign. If they had been given dried shoe leather and it was described as a healing herb, they would have undoubtedly reported fewer illnesses. It doesn't matter how many people were involved: The power of suggestion could be expected to work in all of them. Without a control group and double-blind design no such study can prove much.

A trial that did use a control group followed 80 women with breast cancer, who were given either *Eleutherococcus* or no treatment.[3] The treated individuals showed a lower incidence of nausea, dizziness, and loss of appetite. Unfortunately, this was not a blinded study. Since treated participants knew they were being treated, and the untreated participants knew they weren't, again it's hard to tell how much of the result was due to the power of suggestion.

Double-Blind Studies

Out of the thousands of studies performed on *Panax ginseng*, there were only eight double-blind trials published up through 1990.[4] Most (but not all) of them concluded that ginseng does produce a positive effect on such parameters as physical performance, mental ability, cholesterol levels, and blood sugar control. However, most of the studies were too tiny to prove much, and none were conducted according to modern scientific standards.[5] The situation is similar with *Eleutherococcus*. Fortunately, there have been a few better performed studies published subsequently.

Immune Stimulation

A recent, properly performed, double-blind placebo-controlled study suggests that *Panax ginseng* can improve immunity.[6] This trial enrolled 227 participants at three medical offices in Milan, Italy. Half were given ginseng at a dosage of 100 mg daily, the other half placebo. Four weeks into the study, all participants received influenza vaccine.

The results showed a significant decline in the frequency of colds and flus in the treated group compared to the placebo group (15 versus 42 cases). Also, antibody measurements in response to the vaccination rose higher in the treated group than in the placebo group.

Diabetes

Another properly performed, double-blind study evaluated the effects of *Panax ginseng* (at dosages of 100 mg or 200 mg daily) on 36 people with non-insulin–dependent diabetes.[7] The results showed improvements in blood sugar control.

Mental Function

A recent study found that *Panax ginseng* can improve some aspects of mental function.[8] Over a period of 2 months, 112 healthy, middle-aged adults were given either ginseng or placebo. The results showed that ginseng improved abstract thinking and reaction time. However, there was no change in memory, concentration, or overall subjective experience between the two groups.

Sports Performance

A double-blind study of 20 athletes over an 8-week period found that a standard *Eleutherococcus* formulation produced no improvement in physical performance.[9]

Putting It All Together

Taken together, the scientific record on ginseng is intriguing but not conclusive. If some of the money spent on animal studies had been used to fund more double-blind studies in humans, we might know a lot more. At the present state of knowledge, it is hard to know whether ginseng is as effective as its mystique would make it seem.

Dosage

The typical recommended daily dosage of *Panax ginseng* is 1 to 2 g of raw herb, or 200 mg daily of an extract standardized to contain 4 to 7% ginsenosides. *Eleutherococcus* is taken at a dosage of 2 to 3 g whole herb or 300 to 400 mg of extract daily.

Ordinarily, a 2- to 3-week period of using ginseng is recommended, followed by a 1- to 2-week "rest" period. Russian tradition suggests that ginseng should not be used by those under 40.

Finally, because *Panax ginseng* is so expensive, many products actually contain very little. Adulteration with other herbs and even caffeine is not unusual.[10]

Safety Issues

The various forms of ginseng appear to be nontoxic, both in the short and long term, according to the results of studies in mice, rats, chickens, and dwarf pigs. Ginseng also does not seem to be carcinogenic.[11,12,13]

Side effects are rare. Occasionally women report menstrual abnormalities and/or breast tenderness when they take ginseng, and overstimulation and insomnia have also been reported. Unconfirmed reports suggest that highly excessive doses of ginseng can raise blood pressure, increase heart rate, and possibly cause other significant effects. Whether some of these cases were actually caused by caffeine mixed in with ginseng remains unclear. Ginseng allergy can also occur, as can allergy to any other substance.

In 1979, an article was published in the *Journal of the American Medical Association* claiming that people can become addicted to ginseng and develop blood pressure elevation, nervousness, sleeplessness, diarrhea, and hypersexuality.[14] This report has since been thoroughly discredited and should no longer be taken seriously.[15,16]

However, there is some evidence that ginseng can interfere with drug metabolism, specifically drugs processed by an enzyme called "CYP 3A4." Ask your physician or pharmacist whether you are taking any medications of this type. There have also been specific reports of ginseng interacting with MAO inhibitor drugs and digitalis, although again it is not clear whether it was the ginseng or a contaminant that caused the problem.

Safety in young children, pregnant or nursing women, or those with severe liver or kidney disease has not been established. Interestingly, Chinese tradition suggests that ginseng should not be used by pregnant or nursing mothers.

GOLDENROD
(SOLIDAGO SPP.)

Principal Proposed Uses

Mild bladder infections, bladder/kidney stones

Goldenrod is often falsely accused of being an intensely allergenic plant, because of its unfortunate tendency to bloom brightly at the same time and often in locations quite near to the truly allergenic ragweed. However, actual allergic reactions to this gorgeous plant are unusual.

There are numerous species of goldenrod (27 have been collected in Indiana alone) but all seem to possess similar medicinal properties, and various species are used interchangeably in Europe.[1]

What Is Goldenrod Used for Today?

In Europe, goldenrod is used as a supportive treatment for bladder infections, irritation of the urinary tract, and bladder/kidney stones. Goldenrod increases the flow of urine, helping to wash out bacteria and kidney stones, and may also directly soothe inflamed tissues and calm muscle spasms in the urinary tract.[2] It isn't used as a cure in itself, but rather as a support to other, more definitive treatments such as antibiotics.

We don't really know how well the herb works. Several studies have found that goldenrod increases urine flow,[3] but there is no direct evidence that the herb is effective in resolving bladder infections or bladder/kidney stones. Its active ingredients are not known.

Warning: Since urinary conditions are potentially serious, seek a doctor's supervision.

Dosage

A typical dosage is 3 to 4 g of dried herb 2 to 3 times daily. Make sure to drink plenty of water while taking goldenrod, to help it do its job.

Safety Issues

The safety of goldenrod hasn't been fully evaluated. However, no significant reactions or side effects have been reported.[4] Safety in young children, pregnant and nursing women, or those with severe liver or kidney disease has not been established.

GOLDENSEAL

(HYDRASTIS CANADENSIS)

Principal Proposed Uses

Topical uses: Poorly healing sores, fungal infections, inflamed mucous membranes

Internal uses: Minor digestive problems, sore throat

Other Proposed Uses

Urinary tract infections

Incorrect Proposed Uses

Masking positive findings on drug screens, "immune stimulant," "antibiotic" for common cold

Although goldenseal root is one of the most popular herbs sold today, it is taken almost entirely for the wrong reasons (see What Is Goldenseal Used for Today?). Originally, it was used by Native Americans both as a dye and as a treatment for skin disorders, digestive problems, liver disease, diarrhea, and eye irritations. European settlers learned of the herb from the Iroquois and other tribes and quickly adopted goldenseal as a part of early colonial medical care.

In the early 1800s, a flamboyant herbalist named Samuel Thompson created a wildly popular system of medicine (some would say personality cult) that swept the country. Thompson spoke of goldenseal in glowing terms, as a nearly magical cure for many conditions. His evangelism led to a dramatic upsurge in demand, followed by overcollection and decimation of the wild plant. Prices skyrocketed and then collapsed when Thompsonianism faded away.

Goldenseal has passed through several more booms and busts. Today, it is again in great demand, but now it is under intentional cultivation.

What Is Goldenseal Used for Today?

Contemporary herbalists use goldenseal primarily as a topical antibiotic for wounds that are not healing well. In practice, goldenseal salves, creams, ointments, and powders appear to speed wound healing.

Unfortunately, there are no reliable scientific studies to verify this strong clinical impression. What we do know is that one of goldenseal's constituents, berberine, possesses strong activity against a wide variety of bacteria and fungi.[1,2] Another factor may be that goldenseal seems to have a soothing effect on inflamed mucous membranes.

Goldenseal is most effective by direct contact. It does not seem to be an effective oral antibiotic, probably because the blood levels of berberine that can be achieved by taking goldenseal orally are far too low to matter.[3] However, goldenseal may also be beneficial in treating sore throats and diseases of the digestive tract because it can contact the affected area directly. Since berberine is concentrated in the bladder, goldenseal may be useful in resolving urinary tract infections. It may be helpful for treating fungal infections of the skin as well.

Strangely, goldenseal is most commonly used inappropriately. Goldenseal is frequently combined with echinacea to be taken as an "immune booster" and "antibiotic" for the prevention and treatment of colds. However, as the noted herbalist Paul Bergner has pointed out, there are three things wrong with this packaging: (1) there is no credible evidence that goldenseal increases immunity; (2) the herb was never used historically as an early treatment for colds; and (3) antibiotics aren't effective against colds anyway.[4] Nevertheless, the echinacea in these products may be helpful (see the discussion under Echinacea).

Tradition suggests that goldenseal may help relieve the clogged sinuses and chest congestion that can linger after the acute phase of a cold, although there is no scientific evidence to turn to.

The other myth that has helped drive the sales of goldenseal is the widespread street belief that it can block a positive drug screen. The origin of this false idea dates back to a work of fiction published in 1900 by a pharmacist and author named John Uri Lloyd. In *Stringtown on the Pike*, Lloyd's most successful novel, a dead man is found to have traces of goldenseal in his stomach. In fact, he had taken goldenseal regularly (and correctly) as a digestive aid, but a toxicology expert mistakes the goldenseal for strychnine, and deduces intentional murder.

This work of fiction sufficed to create a folkloric connection between goldenseal and drug testing. Although the goldenseal in the story actually made a drug test come out falsely positive, this has been turned around to become a belief that goldenseal can make urine drug screens come out negative. A word to the wise: It doesn't work.

Dosage

When used as a topical for skin wounds, a sufficient quantity of goldenseal cream, ointment, or powder should be applied to cover the wound. Make sure to clean the wound at least once a day to prevent goldenseal particles from being trapped in the healing tissues.

For mouth sores and sore throats, goldenseal tincture may be swished or gargled. Goldenseal may also be used as strong tea for this purpose, made by boiling 0.5 to 1 g in a cup of water. Goldenseal tea can also be used as a douche for vaginal candidiasis.

For oral use, to aid the digestive tract or loosen clogged sinuses, a typical dosage of goldenseal is 250 to 500 mg 3 times daily. Goldenseal is generally only taken for a couple of weeks at most.

Safety Issues

Goldenseal appears to be safe when used as directed. One widespread rumor claims that goldenseal can disrupt the normal bacteria of the intestines. However, there is no scientific evidence that this occurs, and many herbalists believe that such concerns are unwarranted.[5] Another fallacy is that small overdoses of goldenseal are toxic, causing ulcerations of the stomach and other mucous membranes. This idea is based on a misunderstanding of old literature.[6]

However, because berberine has been reported to cause uterine contractions in animals, goldenseal should not be taken by pregnant women.[7] Safety in young children, nursing women, or those with severe liver or kidney disease is also not established.

Side effects of oral goldenseal are uncommon, although there have been reports of gastrointestinal distress and increased nervousness in people who take very high doses.

GOTU KOLA

(CENTELLA ASIATICA)

Principal Proposed Uses

Varicose veins

Other Proposed Uses

Hemorrhoids, keloid scars, scleroderma, burn and wound healing, improving mental performance

---

Gotu kola is a creeping plant native to subtropical and tropical climates. In India and Indonesia, gotu kola has a long history of use to promote wound healing and slow the progress of leprosy. It was also reputed to prolong life, increase energy, and enhance sexual potency.[1] Other uses of gotu kola included treating skin diseases, diarrhea, menstrual disorders, vaginal discharge, and venereal disease.

Based on these many traditional indications, gotu kola was accepted as a drug in France in the 1880s. British physicians in Africa used a special extract to treat leprosy.

What Is Gotu Kola Used for Today?

In the 1970s, Italian and other European researchers found evidence that gotu kola could significantly improve symptoms of varicose veins, particularly overall discomfort, tiredness, and swelling. However, the herb is not believed to do much to reduce the unsightliness of veins that are already badly damaged. Some clinicians suggest that regular use of gotu kola can prevent the development of visible varicose veins, but this hasn't been proven. Gotu kola has also been suggested as a treatment for hemorrhoids because they are a type of varicose vein.

Like other herbs used for the treatment of varicose veins, gotu kola appears to have a generally beneficial effect on connective tissues. Along these lines, it has been used to prevent the development of keloid (bulging, enlarged) scars following surgery, as well as to soften existing keloids. Gotu kola has also been tried as a treatment for improving burn and wound healing and to alleviate the symptoms of the connective tissue disease scleroderma.

Gotu kola has a reputation for improving memory, and the positive results from a study of rats performed in 1992 produced a temporary rush of public interest.[2] However, the benefits in humans, if any, are far from impressive.

Gotu kola should not be confused with the caffeine-containing kola nut, used in original recipes for Coca Cola.

What Is the Scientific Evidence for Gotu Kola?

Several small-to-moderate double-blind studies suggest that gotu kola is an effective treatment for vein problems of the legs.[3] One followed 87 people divided into three groups: a placebo group and two others, which received either 30 or 60 mg of a standard gotu kola extract twice a day respectively.[4] The results showed improvements in both treated groups, but researchers saw more improvement in those who were treated with the higher dose. This kind of "dose responsiveness" tends to be a strong indicator that a treatment is really working.

Although the subject is far from completely understood, it appears that gotu kola may improve the structure and function of the connective tissue in the body, keeping veins stronger and also possibly reducing the symptoms of other connective-tissue diseases. Along these lines, numerous clinical reports and uncontrolled studies suggest that gotu kola extracts may be useful in treating keloids, burns, wounds, anal fissures, bladder ulcers, dermatitis, fibrocystic breast disease, hemorrhoids, perineal lesions, periodontal disease, cellulite, liver cirrhosis and scleroderma.[5] While some of these studies are intriguing and make a good case for further research, none can be regarded as definitive.

Dosage

The usual dosage of gotu kola is 20 to 40 mg 3 times daily of an extract standardized to contain 40% asiaticoside, 29 to 30% asiatic acid, 29 to 30% madecassic acid, and 1 to 2% madecassoside. Be patient, because gotu kola takes at least 4 weeks to work.

For the prevention of keloid scars, the herb is usually taken for 3 months prior to surgery, and for another 3 months afterwards.

Safety Issues

Orally, gotu kola appears to be nontoxic.[6] It seldom causes any side effects other than the occasional allergic skin rash. However, there are some concerns that gotu kola may be carcinogenic if applied topically to the skin.[7]

Although gotu kola has not been proven safe for pregnant or nursing women, studies in rabbits suggest that it does not harm fetal development,[8] and pregnant women were enrolled in one research trial.[9] Safety in young children and those with severe liver or kidney disease has not been established.

GRAPE SEED PCOs

Principal Proposed Uses

Strengthening blood vessels and reducing inflammation (e.g., varicose veins, hemorrhoids, swelling after injury or surgery, easy bruising)

Other Proposed Uses

Poor night vision, aging skin, macular degeneration, cancer (prevention), diabetic neuropathy, allergies, atherosclerosis (prevention), diabetic retinopathy, heart disease (prevention)

One of the best-selling herbal products of the early 1990s was an extract of the bark of French maritime pine. This substance consists of a family of chemicals known scientifically as procyanidolic oligomers (PCOs) or oligomeric proanthycyanadin complexes (OPCs). Similar substances are also found in grape seed.

The modern use of PCOs is closely linked to an event in 1534, when a French explorer and his crew were trapped by ice in the Saint Lawrence River. Many of the men were saved from scurvy by a Native American who suggested they make tea from the needles and bark of a local pine tree. Over 400 years later, Jacques Masquelier of the University of Bordeaux came across this story and decided to investigate the constituents of pine trees. In 1951, he extracted PCOs from the bark of the maritime pine, and found that it could duplicate many of the functions of vitamin C. Later, he found an even better source of PCOs in grape seed, which is their major source in France today.

Like bilberry anthocyanosides (to which they are closely related), PCOs appear to stabilize the walls of blood vessels, reduce inflammation, and generally support tissues containing collagen.[1-4] PCOs are also strong antioxidants. Vitamin E defends against fat-soluble oxidants and vitamin C neutralizes water-soluble ones, but PCOs are active against both types.[5,6,7]

What Are Grape Seed PCOs Used for Today?

In Europe, grape seed PCOs are widely used to treat conditions in which blood vessels are weakened, damaged, or inflamed, such as varicose veins, easy bruising, and hemmorrhoids. Leakage from inflamed and damaged blood vessels is also a major cause of swelling in injured tissues. For this reason, PCOs are also used to reduce swelling caused by surgery or sports injuries.

PCOs are also sometimes recommended to restore aging skin on the theory that they can help restore damaged collagen and to reduce symptoms of allergies on the grounds that allergic reactions involve inflammation. Like bilberry, PCOs are also used for impaired night vision. Finally, just as with other antioxidants, regular use of PCOs has been proposed to prevent or treat atherosclerosis, cancer, diabetic retinopathy, diabetic neuropathy, and macular degeneration.

What Is the Scientific Evidence for Grape Seed PCOs?

There appear to be about 13 double-blind studies of PCOs. However, they were published in French, and few have been translated into English.

Varicose Veins (Venous Insufficiency)

A double-blind study compared PCOs against placebo in 92 participants, showing improvement in 75% of the treated group as compared to 41% in the control group.[8] According to sketchy information provided by one manufacturer, a controlled study of 291 individuals with varicose veins also found significant benefit.[9] Finally, a double-blind study of 50 people with varicose veins of the legs found that doses of 150 mg per day of PCOs were more effective in reducing symptoms and signs than another natural treatment: the bioflavonoid diosmin, widely used in Europe for this condition.[10]

Edema

Breast cancer surgery often leads to swelling of the arm. A double-blind placebo-controlled study of 63 post-operative breast cancer patients found that 600 mg of PCOs daily for 6 months reduced edema, pain, and peculiar sensations known as paresthesias.[11] Also, in a double-blind placebo-controlled study of 32 "face-lift" patients who were followed for 10 days, edema disappeared much faster in the treated group.[12]

Another 10-day double-blind placebo-controlled study enrolling 50 participants found that PCOs improved the rate at which edema disappeared following sports injuries.[13]

Night Vision

One interesting 6-week study evaluated the ability of grape seed extract to improve night vision in normal subjects.[14,15] In this trial of 100 healthy volunteers, those who received 200 mg per day of PCOs showed improvements in night vision and glare recovery as compared to placebo-treated subjects.

Atherosclerosis

Although there are no reliable human studies, animal evidence suggests that PCOs can slow or reverse atherosclerosis.[16–19] This suggests that PCOs might be helpful for preventing heart disease.

Dosage

For use as a general antioxidant (much as you might use vitamin E or vitamin C), 50 mg of PCOs daily are sufficient. A higher dosage of 150 to 300 mg daily is generally used for treating specific diseases such as varicose veins. Grape seed PCOs are just as good and much less expensive than the maritime pine source.

Safety Issues

Extensive studies have found PCOs to be nontoxic.[20] Side effects are rare and limited to mild gastrointestinal distress. However, safety in young children, pregnant or nursing women, or those with severe liver or kidney disease has not been conclusively established.

GREEN TEA
(CAMELLIA SINENSIS)

Principal Proposed Uses

Cancer prevention

People have been drinking tea for thousands of years, but only in the last couple of decades have we begun to document the potential health benefits of this ancient beverage. Both black and green tea are made from the same plant, but more of the original substances endure in the less-processed green form. Green tea contains high levels of substances called polyphenols, known to possess strong antioxidant, anticarcinogenic, and even antibiotic properties.[1]

A growing body of evidence in both human and animal studies suggests that regular consumption of green tea can reduce the incidence of a variety of cancers, including colon, pancreatic, and stomach cancers.[2] However, the observational studies used to draw these conclusions can be misleading, and not everyone who examines the data concludes that green tea has been proven effective.[3]

What Is Green Tea Used for Today?

Based on the widely publicized results of the observational studies mentioned earlier, green tea has become popular as a daily drink for cancer prevention. (For more information on cancer prevention, see *The Natural Pharmacist Guide to Reducing Cancer Risk.*)

Dosage

Studies suggest that 3 cups of green tea daily provides protection against cancer. However, because not everyone wants to take the time to drink green tea, manufacturers have offered extracts that can be taken in pill form. A typical dosage is 100 to 150 mg 3 times daily of a green tea extract standardized to contain 80% total polyphenols and 50% epigallocatechin gallate. Whether these extracts work as well as the real thing remains unknown.

Safety Issues

As a widely consumed beverage, green tea is generally regarded as safe. It does contain caffeine, although at a lower level than black tea or coffee, and can therefore cause insomnia, nervousness, and the other well-known symptoms of excess caffeine intake. Green tea should not be given to infants and young children.

GUGGUL
(COMMIPHORA MUKUL)

Principal Proposed Uses
High cholesterol

Guggul, the sticky gum resin from the mukul myrrh tree, plays a major role in the traditional herbal medicine of India. It was traditionally combined with other herbs for the treatment of arthritis, skin diseases, pains in the nervous system, obesity, digestive problems, infections in the mouth, and menstrual problems.

In the early 1960s, Indian researchers discovered an ancient Sanskrit medical text that appears to clearly describe the symptoms and treatment of high cholesterol.[1] One of the main recommendations was guggul. Subsequent tests in animals found that guggul gum both lowered cholesterol levels and also separately protected against the development of hardening of the arteries.

Numerous research trials followed this discovery, culminating in open and double-blind studies examining guggul's effectiveness in humans.[2,3] Although these studies showed positive results, they are small and have real problems in scientific design, making the results less than definitive. Nonetheless, the evidence was strong enough for the Indian government to approve guggul as a treatment for high cholesterol.

What Is Guggul Used for Today?

It appears that guggul can lower cholesterol by about 11% and triglycerides by 17%, as well as raise HDL (good) cholesterol levels and lower LDL (bad) cholesterol levels.[4,5] The full benefits take about 4 weeks to develop.

Dosage

Take a dose of guggul extract standardized to provide 25 mg of gugulsterone 3 times daily. For best results in lowering cholesterol, increase exercise and improve diet as well. (See *The Natural Pharmacist Guide to Garlic and Cholesterol* for more information on guggul and other natural treatments to lower cholesterol.)

Safety Issues

Guggul appears to be reasonably safe, but thorough safety studies have not yet been performed.[6,7] Whole-gum guggul can cause digestive distress. However, extracts standardized to gugulsterone content seldom cause significant immediate problems.

Safety in young children, pregnant or nursing women, or those with severe liver or kidney disease has not been established.

GYMNEMA
(GYMNEMA SYLVESTRE)

Principal Proposed Uses
Diabetes (blood sugar control)

Native to the forests of India, *Gymnema sylvestre* has a coincidental double relationship to sugar: When placed on the tongue, it blocks the sensation of sweetness, and when taken internally, it appears to help control blood sugar levels in diabetes. There doesn't seem to be any connection between these two effects.

Indian physicians first used gymnema to treat diabetes almost 2,000 years ago. In the 1920s, preliminary scientific studies found that gymnema leaves do indeed reduce blood sugar levels,[1] but nothing much came of this discovery for decades.

What Is Gymnema Used for Today?

With the recent revival of interest in herbs, gymnema has become increasingly popular in the United States as a supportive treatment for diabetes. A few animal and preliminary human studies suggest that gymnema can increase insulin secretion and also enhance insulin's effectiveness.[2,3,4] Gymnema is most likely to be helpful in mild cases of adult-onset diabetes when insulin injections are not yet required. However, it is also used as a supportive treatment in more serious forms of the disease. (For more information on diabetes, see *The Natural Pharmacist Guide to Diabetes*.)

Warning: Diabetes is a dangerous illness, thus gymnema should only be used under medical supervision. Under no circumstances should you try to replace insulin with gymnema alone.

Dosage

Gymnema is usually taken at a dosage of 400 to 600 mg daily of an extract standardized to contain 24% gymnemic acid.

Safety Issues

When used in appropriate dosages, gymnema appears to be fairly safe, although extensive studies have not been performed. One obvious risk is that if gymnema is successful, it may lower blood sugar levels too far, causing a dangerous hypoglycemic reaction. For this reason, medical supervision is essential.

Safety in young children, pregnant or nursing women, or those with severe kidney or liver disease has not been established.

HAWTHORN

(CRATAEGUS OXYACANTHA)

Principal Proposed Uses

Early stages of congestive heart failure, benign heart palpitations, high blood pressure

The name "hawthorn" is derived from "hedgethorn," reflecting this spiny tree's use as a living fence in much of Europe. Besides protecting estates from trespassers, hawthorn has also been used medicinally since ancient times. Roman physicians used hawthorn as a heart drug in the first century A.D., but most of the literature from that period focuses on its symbolic use for religious rites and political ceremonies.

During the Middle Ages, hawthorn was used for the treatment of dropsy, a condition we now call congestive heart failure. It was also used for treating other heart ailments as well as for sore throat.

What Is Hawthorn Used for Today?

Hawthorn is widely regarded in modern Europe as a safe and effective treatment for the early stages of congestive heart failure. Although not as potent as that other famous heart herb of the Middle Ages, foxglove, hawthorn is much safer. The active ingredients in foxglove are the drugs digoxin and digitoxin. However, hawthorn does not appear to have any single active ingredient. This has prevented it from being turned into a drug.

Like foxglove and the drugs made from it, hawthorn appears to improve the heart's pumping ability. But it offers one very important advantage. Digitalis and some other medications that increase the power of the heart also make it more irritable and liable to dangerous irregularities of rhythm. In contrast, hawthorn has the unique property of both strengthening the heart and stabilizing it against arrythmias by lengthening what is called the *refractory period*.[1,2,3] This term refers to the short period following a heartbeat during which the heart cannot beat again. Many irregularities of heart rhythm begin with an early beat. Digitalis shortens the refractory period, making such a premature beat more likely, while hawthorn protects against such potentially dangerous breaks in the heart's even rhythm. Also, with digitalis the difference between the proper dosage and the toxic dosage is very small. Hawthorn has an enormous range of safe dosing.[4]

Nevertheless, I don't recommend self-treating congestive heart failure! The disease is simply too dangerous. There are also medical treatments (such as ACE inhibitors) that have been proven to save lives in CHF, a benefit that hawthorn may not provide. You need a physician versed in both conventional and alternative medicine to guide you if you wish to use hawthorn for this condition.

There is one condition in which you may be able to safely use hawthorn as a self-treatment: annoying heart palpitations that have been thoroughly evaluated and found to be benign. Common symptoms include occasional thumping as well as episodes of racing heartbeat. These may occur without any identifiable medical cause and may not require any medical treatment, except for purposes of comfort. Although there is little scientific evidence to support it, many people use hawthorn for this condition.

However, because there are many dangerous kinds of heart palpitations, it is absolutely necessary to get a thorough checkup first. You should only self-treat with hawthorn after a doctor tells you that you have no medically significant heart problems. Full benefits may take a month or two to develop.

Finally, hawthorn sometimes lowers blood pressure a little, but seldom enough to make a significant difference.[5,6]

What Is the Scientific Evidence for Hawthorn?

There has been a significant amount of solid research regarding the use of hawthorn as a treatment for congestive heart failure. Between 1981 and 1994, 13 controlled clinical studies of hawthorn were performed, most of them double-blind.[7,8] In all, 808 people participated in these trials. The cumulative results strongly suggest that hawthorn is an effective treatment for congestive heart failure. Comparative studies suggest that hawthorn is about as effective as a low dose of the conventional drug captopril, although whether it produces the same long-term benefits as captopril is unknown.[9]

Dosage

The standard dosage of hawthorn is 100 to 300 mg 3 times daily of an extract standardized to contain about 2 to 3% flavonoids or 18 to 20% procyanidins. Full effects appear to take several weeks or months to develop.

Safety Issues

Hawthorn appears to be safe. Germany's Commission E lists no known risks, contraindications, or drug interactions with hawthorn, and mice and rats have been given phenomenal doses without showing significant toxicity.[10] However, since hawthorn affects the heart, it shouldn't be combined with other heart drugs without a doctor's supervision. People with especially low blood pressure should also exercise caution.

Side effects are rare, mostly consisting of mild stomach upset and occasional allergic reactions (skin rash).

Safety in young children, pregnant or nursing women, or those with severe liver, heart or kidney disease has not been established.

HE SHOU WU a.k.a. FO TI
(POLYGONUM MULTIFLORUM)

Principal Proposed Uses

High cholesterol, insomnia, constipation

The name of this herb literally means "Black-haired Mr. He," in reference to an ancient story of a Mr. He who restored his vitality, sexual potency, and youthful appearance by taking the herb now named after him. He shou wu is widely used in China for the traditional purpose of restoring black hair and other signs of youth.

More so than with most Chinese herbs, tradition supports taking He shou wu as a single herb, although it also figures as a component in many formulas. He shou wu is also called fo ti; pure unprocessed root is named white fo ti, while herb boiled in black-bean liquid according to a traditional process is called red fo ti. The two forms are believed to have somewhat different properties.

What Is He Shou Wu Used for Today?

Both animal and preliminary human studies performed in China suggest that He shou wu can reduce serum cholesterol and also improve symptoms of insomnia.[1]

He shou wu is also said to be useful for constipation; although if this is true, the effect is mild.

I tried He shou wu to see if it would turn my graying hair black, but nothing happened. Based on this highly sophisticated scientific research, I suspect that Mr. He's experience is hard to duplicate. (But then again, anecdotal negative data is just as bad as anecdotal positive data!)

Dosage

He shou wu should be taken at a dosage of 9 to 15 g of raw herb per day, or according to the label for processed extracts. For most purposes, the processed or "red" fo ti is said to be superior. However, the raw herb is believed to be more effective for relieving constipation.

Safety Issues

Detailed modern safety studies have not been performed on this herb. Immediate side effects are infrequent, primarily limited to mild diarrhea and the rare allergic reaction. Safety for young children, pregnant or nursing women, or those with severe kidney or liver disease has not been established.

HOPS

(HUMULUS LUPULUS)

Principal Proposed Uses

Anxiety, insomnia, digestive problems

Hops (the fruiting bodies of the hop plant) are most famous as the source of beer's bitter flavor, but they have a long history of use in herbal medicine as well. In Greece and Rome, hops were used as a remedy for poor digestion and intestinal disturbances. The Chinese used the herb for these purposes as well as to treat leprosy and tuberculosis.

As cultivation of hops for beer spread through Europe, it gradually became obvious that workers in hop fields tended to fall asleep on the job, more so than could be explained by the tedium of the work. This observation led to enthusiasm for using hops as a sedative. However, subsequent investigation suggests that much of the sedative effect seen in hop fields is due to an oil that evaporates quickly in storage.

Despite the absence of this oil, dried hop preparations do appear to be somewhat calming. While the exact reason is not clear, it seems that a sedating substance known as methylbutenol develops in the dried herb over a period of time.[1] It may also be manufactured in the body from other constituents of dried hops.

What Are Hops Used for Today?

Germany's Commission E authorizes the use of hops for "discomfort due to restlessness or anxiety and sleep disturbances." Because its sedative effect is mild at most, the herb is often combined with other treatments.

Like other bitter plants, hops are also used to improve appetite and digestion.

Scientists have had difficulty demonstrating that hops cause sedation.[2]

Dosage

The standard dosage of hops is 0.5 g taken 1 to 3 times daily.

Safety Issues

Hops are believed to be nontoxic. However, as with all herbs, some people are allergic to it. Interestingly, some species of dogs, greyhounds in particular, appear to be sensitive to hops with reports of deaths occurring.[3] The mechanism of this toxicity is not yet known. Those taken with the popular hobby of brewing beer at home are advised to keep pets away from the relatively large quantity of hops used in this process.

HORSE CHESTNUT

(AESCULUS HIPPOCASTANUM)

Principal Proposed Uses

Vein problems (e.g., varicose veins, phlebitis, hemorrhoids)

Other Proposed Uses

Swelling (sprains and other injuries)

The horse chestnut tree is widely cultivated for its bright white, yellow, or red flower clusters. Closely related to the Ohio buckeye, its spiny fruits contain a few large seeds known as horse chestnuts. A superstition in many parts of Europe suggests that carrying these seeds in your pocket will ward off rheumatism. More serious medical uses date back to nineteenth-century France, where extracts were used to treat hemorrhoids.

What Is Horse Chestnut Used for Today?

Serious German research began in the 1960s and ultimately led to the approval of an extract of horse chestnut for vein diseases of the legs. This herb is the third most common single herb product sold in Germany, after ginkgo and St. John's wort. In Japan, an injectable form of horse chestnut is widely used to reduce inflammation after surgery or injury, however it is not available in the United States.

The active ingredients in horse chestnut appear to be a group of chemicals called saponins, of which aescin is considered the most important. Like PCOs and bilberry, aescin has the capacity to reduce swelling and inflammation, probably by slowing down the rate at which fluid leaks from irritated capillaries.[1] It's not exactly clear how aescin works, but theories include "sealing" leaking capillaries, improving the elastic strength of veins, and preventing the release of enzymes (known as glycosaminoglycan hydrolases) that break down collagen and open holes in capillary walls.[2]

Horse chestnut is most often used as a treatment for venous insufficiency. This is a condition associated with varicose veins, when the blood pools in the veins of the leg and causes aching, swelling, and a sense of heaviness. While horse chestnut appears to reduce these symptoms, it is not believed to improve visible varicose veins very much.

Because hemorrhoids are actually a form of varicose veins, horse chestnut is often recommended for them as well.

Based on its known effects on veins, horse chestnut is also sometimes used along with conventional treatment in cases where the veins of the lower legs become seriously inflamed (phlebitis). However, this condition is potentially dangerous and requires a doctor's supervision.

Just like PCOs, extracts of horse chestnut are sometimes recommended to help reduce swelling after sprains and other athletic injuries. Again, this use is based on the known effects of horse chestnut on blood vessels.

What Is the Scientific Evidence for Horse Chestnut?

A total of 558 individuals have been involved in double-blind studies of horse chestnut for treating venous insufficiency.[3] One of the largest trials followed 212 people over a period of 40 days.[4] It was what is called a *crossover study* because the participants initially received horse chestnut or placebo, and then they were crossed over to the other treatment (without their knowledge) after 20 days. The results showed that horse chestnut produced significant improvement in leg edema, pain, and sensation of heaviness.

Another study compared the effectiveness of horse chestnut and compression stockings in 240 people over a course of 12 weeks.[5] Compression stockings worked faster at reducing swelling, but by 12 weeks the results were equivalent.

Dosage

The most common dosage of horse chestnut is 300 mg twice daily standardized to contain 50 mg aescin per dose, for a total daily dose of 100 mg aescin. After good results have been achieved, the dosage can be reduced by about half for maintenance.

Horse chestnut preparations should certify that esculin has been removed. Also, a delayed-release formulation must be used to prevent gastrointestinal upset.

Warning: Do not try to inject horse chestnut products designed for oral use!

Safety Issues

After decades of wide usage in Germany, there have been no reports of harmful effects due to horse chestnut, even when it has been taken in overdose.[6] In animal studies, horse chestnut and its principal ingredient aescin have been found to be very safe, even when taken at dosages seven times higher than normal. Dogs and rats have been treated for 34 weeks with this herb without harmful effects.[7] However, dosages 50 times higher than normal can cause death in animals, and in Japan, where injectable forms are used, dangerous and even fatal reactions have been noted.[8]

For theoretical reasons, horse chestnut is not recommended for people with serious kidney or liver disease. It also should not be combined with anticoagulant or "blood-thinning" drugs, as it may alter their function.

The safety of horse chestnut in young children, and pregnant or nursing women has not been established. However, 13 pregnant women were given horse chestnut in a controlled study without noticeable harm.[9]

In clinical studies of horse chestnut, there have been no significant side effects other than the usual occasional mild allergic reactions or gastrointestinal distress. However, these studied all used controlled-release forms of horse chestnut. Taking this herb in other formulations may cause quite a bit of stomach upset.

HORSETAIL

(EQUISETUM ARVENSE)

Principal Proposed Uses

Brittle nails, osteoporosis, rheumatoid arthritis

Horsetail is a living fossil, the sole descendent of primitive plants that served as dinosaur snacks 100 million years ago. The herb is unique for its high concentration of silicon, as well as for its ability to dissolve gold and other minerals into itself. Because of its silicon content, horsetail is abrasive enough to be used for polishing.

Medicinally, horsetail has been used for treating urinary disorders, wounds, gonorrhea, nosebleeds, digestive disorders, gout, and many other conditions.[1]

What Is Horsetail Used for Today?

Silicon plays a role in bone health, and for this reason, horsetail has been recommended to keep bones and nails strong.[2] The famous German herbalist Rudolf Weiss also suggests that horsetail can relieve symptoms of rheumatoid arthritis.[3] However, there is no real scientific evidence for any of these uses.

Dosage

The standard dosage of horsetail is 1 g in capsule or tea form up to 3 times daily, as needed. Medicinal horsetail should *not* be confused with its highly toxic relative, the marsh horsetail *(Equisetum palustre)*.

Safety Issues

Noticeable side effects from standard dosages of horsetail tea are rare. However, horsetail contains an enzyme that damages the vitamin thiamine and has caused severe illness and even death in livestock that consumed too much of it.[4] In Canada, horsetail products are required to undergo heating or other forms of processing to inactivate this harmful constituent.

Also, perhaps because horsetail contains low levels of nicotine, children have been known to become seriously ill from using the branches as blow guns.[5] This plant can also concentrate toxic metals present in its environment.

For all of the above reasons, horsetail is not recommended for young children, pregnant or nursing women, or those with severe kidney or liver disease.

JUNIPER

(JUNIPERIS COMMUNIS)

Principal Proposed Uses

Bladder infections

In Dutch, juniper is called "geniver," from which came the name "gin." But juniper is not only good for making martinis. Its berries (actually not berries at all, but a portion of the cone) were used by the Zuni Indians to assist in childbirth, by British herbalists to treat congestive heart failure and stimulate menstruation, and by American nineteenth-century herbalists to treat congestive heart failure, gonorrhea, and urinary tract infections.

The explanation for some of these uses may be found in juniper's diuretic properties. Its volatile oils have been shown to increase the rate of kidney filtration,[1] thereby perhaps helping to remove the accumulated fluid in congestive heart failure, and "wash out" the offending bacteria in urinary tract infections. However, there is no direct scientific evidence that juniper is effective for these purposes.

What Is Juniper Used for Today?

Contemporary herbalists primarily use juniper as a component of herbal formulas designed to treat bladder infections. A typical combination might include uva ursi, parsley, cleavers, and buchu. Such formulas are said to be most effective when taken at the first sign of symptoms and may not work well once the infection has really taken hold. Unfortunately, double-blind studies of juniper have not been performed.

Recently, gin-soaked raisins have been touted as an arthritis treatment. This is probably just a fad, but some weak evidence suggests that juniper may possess antiinflammatory properties.[2] In the test tube, juniper has also been shown to inhibit herpes virus.[3]

Dosage

You can make juniper tea by adding 1 cup of boiling water to 1 tablespoon of juniper berries, covering, and allowing the berries to steep for 20 minutes. The usual dosage is 1 cup twice a day. However, juniper is said to work better as a treatment for bladder infections when combined with other herbs. Combination products should be taken according to label instructions.

Warning: Bladder infections can go on to become kidney infections. For this reason, seek medical supervision if your symptoms don't resolve in a few days, or if you develop intense low back pain, fever, chills, or other signs of serious infection.

Safety Issues

Although juniper is regarded as safe and is widely used in foods, I don't recommend taking it during pregnancy. (I also recommend not drinking gin.) Remember, juniper was used historically to stimulate menstruation and childbirth. It has also been shown to cause miscarriages in rats.[4]

Juniper seldom causes any noticeable side effects. Prolonged use of juniper could possibly deplete the body of potassium, the way other diuretics do, but this hasn't been proven. Combining juniper with conventional diuretics, however, may cause excessive fluid loss.

Some texts warn that juniper oil may be a kidney irritant, but there is no real evidence that this is the case.[5] Nonetheless, people with serious kidney disease probably shouldn't take juniper. Safety for young children, nursing women, or those with severe liver disease has also not been established.

KAVA
(PIPER METHYSTICUM)

Principal Proposed Uses
Anxiety, insomnia

Other Proposed Uses
Alcohol withdrawal, tension headaches

Kava is a member of the pepper family that has long been cultivated by Pacific Islanders for use as a social and ceremonial drink. The first description of kava came to the West from Captain James Cook on his celebrated voyages through the South Seas. Cook reported that on occasions when village elders and chieftains gathered together for significant meetings, they would hold an elaborate kava ceremony at the beginning to break the ice (if there's any ice in the South Seas). Typically, each participant would drink two or three bowls of chewed-up kava mixed with coconut milk. Kava was also drunk in less formal social settings as a mild intoxicant.

When they learned about kava's effects, European scientists set to work trying to isolate its active ingredients. However, it wasn't until 1966 that substances named kavalactones were isolated and found to be effective sedatives. One of the most active of these is dihydrokavain, which has been found to produce a sedative, painkilling, and anticonvulsant effect.[1,2,3] Other named kavalactones include kavain, methysticin, and dihydromethysticin.

High dosages of kava extracts cause muscular relaxation, and at very high dosages paralysis without loss of consciousness develops.[4-7] Kava is also a local anesthetic, producing peculiar numbing sensations when held in the mouth.

The method of action of kava is not fully understood. Conventional tranquilizers in the valium family interact with special binding sites in the brain called GABA receptors. Early studies of kava suggested that the herb does not affect these receptors.[8] However, more recent studies have found an interaction.[9] The early researchers may have missed the connection because kava appears to affect somewhat unusual parts of the brain.

What Is Kava Used for Today?

In the words of Germany's Commission E, kava is useful for relieving "states of nervous anxiety, tension, and agitation." While it is not considered powerful enough to treat severe anxiety or panic attacks, kava is often used for milder symptoms. Its skeletal-muscle relaxing effects may make it particularly useful if you suffer from tension headaches. While prescription drugs for anxiety are generally more powerful, kava does not seem to impair mental functioning.[10,11]

The Commission E monograph recommends using kava for no more than 3 months, and accompanying its use with more curative treatments such as psychotherapy.

Warning: Various medical conditions, such as hyperthyroidism, can produce symptoms similar to anxiety. Medical evaluation is strongly recommended before self-treating with kava.

There is some evidence that kava can help insomnia.[12] It has also been proposed as a treatment for tension headaches and as an aid to alcohol withdrawal. (For more information on kava, see *The Natural Pharmacist Guide to Kava and Anxiety*.)

What Is the Scientific Evidence for Kava?

There have been five meaningful studies of kava, involving a total of about 400 participants. The best of these was a 6-month double-blind study that tested kava's effectiveness in 100 people with various forms of anxiety.[13] Over the course of the trial, they were evaluated with a list of questions called the Hamilton Anxiety Scale (HAM-A). The HAM-A assigns a total score based on such symptoms as restlessness, nervousness, heart palpitations, stomach discomfort, dizziness, and chest pain. Lower scores indicate reduced anxiety. Participants who were given kava showed significantly improved scores beginning at 8 weeks and continuing throughout the duration of the treatment.

This study is notable for the long delay before kava was effective. Previous studies had showed a good response in 1 week.[14,15,16] The reason for this discrepancy is unclear.

Besides these placebo-controlled studies, one 6-month, double-blind study compared kava against two standard anxiety drugs (oxazepam and brozamepam) in 174 people with anxiety symptoms.[17] Improvement in HAM-A scores was about the same in all groups. However, physicians who use kava state that prescription treatments are usually more powerful in real life. The HAM-A rating scale can only roughly document changes in mood and may not always be able to distinguish between excellent and modest improvement.

Dosage

Kava is usually sold in a standardized form where the total amount of kavalactones per pill is listed. For use as an anti-anxiety agent, the dose of kava should supply about 40 to 70 mg of kavalactones 3 times daily. The total daily dosage should not exceed 300 mg. People who use kava frequently report that effects begin to be obvious in a week or less, but that full benefits require 4 to 8 weeks to manifest.

The proper dosage for insomnia is 210 mg of kavalactones 1 hour before bedtime.

Safety Issues

When used appropriately, kava appears to be safe. Animal studies have shown that dosages of up to four times that of normal cause no problems at all, and 13 times the normal dosage causes only mild problems in rats.[18]

A study of 4,049 people who took a rather low dose of kava (70 mg of kavalactones daily) for 7 weeks found side effects in 1.5% of cases. These were mostly mild gastrointestinal complaints and allergic rashes.[19] A 4-week study of 3,029 individuals given 240 mg of kavalactones daily showed a 2.3% incidence of basically the same side effects.[20] However, long-term use (months to years) of kava in excess of 400 mg kavalactones per day can create a distinctive generalized dry, scaly rash.[21] It disappears promptly when the kava use stops.

Kava does not appear to produce mental cloudiness.[22,23,24] Nonetheless, I wouldn't recommend driving after using kava until you discover how strongly it affects you. It makes some people quite drowsy.

Contrary to many reports in the media, there is no evidence that kava actually improves mental function. Two studies are commonly cited as if to prove this, but actually there was only one study performed: It was described in two separate articles.[25,26] This tiny study found that kava does not impair mental function; however, it doesn't show that kava improves it. A slight improvement *was* seen on a couple of tests, but it was statistically insignificant (too small to mean anything).

High doses of kava are known to cause inebriation. For this reason, there is some concern that it could become an herb of abuse. There have been reports of young people trying to get high by taking products they thought contained kava. One of these products, fX, turned out to contain dangerous drugs but no kava at all. European physicians have not reported any problems with kava addiction.[27] However, one study in mice suggests that it might be possible.[28]

The German Commission E monograph warns against the use of kava during pregnancy and nursing.

Kava should not be taken along with alcohol, prescription tranquilizers or sedatives, or other depressant drugs as there have been reports of coma caused by such combinations.[29] Safety in young children and those with severe liver or kidney disease has not been established.

Transitioning from Medications to Kava

If you're taking Xanax or other drugs in the benzodiazepine family, switching to kava will be very hard. You must seek a doctor's supervision, because withdrawal symptoms can be severe and even life-threatening.

It's easier to make the switch from milder antianxiety drugs, such as BuSpar and antidepressants. Nonetheless, a doctor's supervision is still strongly advised.

KUDZU

(PUERARIA LOBATA)

Principal Proposed Uses

Alcoholism

Other Proposed Uses

Cold with pain in the neck

Kudzu is cooked as food in China, and also is used as an herb in traditional Chinese medicine. However, in the United States, kudzu has become an invasive pest. It was deliberately planted earlier this century for use as animal fodder and to control soil erosion. It turned out to be incredibly prolific and soon spread throughout the South like an alien invader. The problem is that kudzu can grow a foot a day during the summer, and as much as 60 feet a year, giving it the folk name "mile-a-minute vine." It swallows telephone poles, chokes trees, and takes over yards. The only defense may be to find a use for it.

What Is Kudzu Used for Today?

Besides cooking with it, feeding it to animals, and weaving baskets out of its rubbery vines, kudzu may also be useful in treating alcoholism. In Chinese folk medicine, a tea brewed from kudzu root is believed to be useful in "sobering up" a drunk. Taking the hint, a 1993 study evaluated the effects of kudzu in a species of hamsters known to enjoy drinking alcohol to intoxication.[1] Ordinarily, if given a choice, the Syrian golden hamster will prefer alcohol to water, but administration of kudzu reversed that preference. This has led to widespread speculation (but no proof thus far) that kudzu may be useful in the treatment of human alcoholism.

The antialcohol effects of kudzu were initially attributed to the presence of the substances daidzin and daidzein, but later research cast doubt on this explanation.[2] At present, we do not how kudzu may work.

In academic Chinese herbology (as opposed to Chinese folk medicine), kudzu is used for other purposes. One classic herbal formula containing kudzu is recommended for the treatment of colds accompanied by pain in the neck, and modern Chinese herbalists frequently use it for this purpose.

Dosage

The standard dosage of kudzu ranges from 9 to 15 g daily, in tea or tablets. The proper length of treatment for alcoholism has not been determined.

Safety Issues

Based on its extensive food use, kudzu is believed to be reasonably safe. However, safety in young children, pregnant or nursing women, or those with severe kidney or liver disease has not been established.

LAPACHO
a.k.a. PAU D'ARCO, TAHEEBO

(TABEBUIA IMPESTIGINOSA)

Principal Proposed Uses

Yeast, respiratory, and bladder infections

Other Proposed Uses

Diarrhea, cancer?

The inner bark of the lapacho tree plays a central role in the herbal medicine of several South American indigenous peoples. They use it to treat cancer as well as a great variety of infectious diseases. There is intriguing, but far from conclusive, scientific evidence for some of these traditional uses. One of lapacho's major ingredients, lapachol, definitely possesses antitumor properties, and for a time was under active investigation as a possible chemotherapy drug. Unfortunately, when given in high enough dosages to kill cancer cells, lapachol causes numerous serious side effects. Another component, b-lapachone, continues to be investigated as an anticancer agent since it may have a better side-effect profile and acts similarly to a new class of prescription antitumor drugs.[1]

Herbalists believe that the whole herb can produce equivalent benefits with fewer side effects, but this claim has never been properly investigated.

Various ingredients in lapacho can also kill bacteria and fungi in the test tube.[2] However, it is not yet clear how well the herb works for this purpose when taken orally.

What Is Lapacho Used for Today?

Based on its traditional use and the fledgling scientific evidence, some herbalists recommend lapacho as a treatment for cancer. However, I do not endorse this usage. There is no good evidence that lapacho is an effective cancer treatment, and cancer is clearly not a disease to trifle with! Furthermore, the mechanism by which lapacho possibly works may cause it to interfere with the action of prescription anticancer drugs. Definitely do not add it to a conventional chemotherapy regime without consulting your physician.

Lapacho is also sometimes used to treat yeast infections, respiratory infections, infectious diarrhea, and bladder infections.

Note: Do not count on lapacho to treat serious infections.

Dosage

Lapacho contains many components that don't dissolve in water, so making tea from the herb is not the best idea. It's better to take capsulized powdered bark, at a standard dosage of 300 mg 3 times daily. For the treatment of yeast and other infections, it is taken until symptoms resolve.

The inner bark of the lapacho tree is believed to be the most effective part of the plant. Unfortunately, inferior products containing only the outer bark and the wood are sometimes misrepresented as "genuine inner-bark lapacho."

Safety Issues

Full safety studies of lapacho have not been performed. When taken in normal dosages, it does not appear to cause any significant side effects.[3] However, because its constituent lapachol is somewhat toxic, the herb is not recommended for pregnant or nursing mothers. Safety in young children or those with severe liver or kidney disease has also not been established.

LICORICE

(GLYCYRRHIZA GLABRA)

Principal Proposed Uses

Oral uses (DGL form): Ulcers, mouth sores, heartburn (esophageal reflux)

Topical uses (whole herb): Eczema, psoriasis, herpes

Oral uses (whole herb): Cough, asthma, chronic fatigue syndrome

A member of the pea family, licorice root has been used since ancient times both as food and as medicine. In Chinese herbology, licorice is an ingredient in nearly all herbal formulas for the traditional purpose of "harmonizing" the separate herbs involved.

Licorice possesses a variety of active ingredients. The most analyzed is glycyrrhizin, which has been found to possess anti-inflammatory, cough-suppressant, antiviral, estrogen-like, and aldosterone-like activities.[1] The natural hormone aldosterone can cause fluid retention, increased blood pressure, and potassium loss. Glycyrrhizin can produce similar effects, which may cause a problem (see the discussion under Safety Issues). To avoid the aldosterone-like effects, manufacturers have found a way to remove glycyrrhizin from licorice, producing the much safer product deglycyrrhizinated licorice, or DGL. However, it is not clear that DGL provides all the same benefits as whole licorice.

What Is Licorice Used for Today?

Licorice appears to have a general healing effect on mucous membranes, perhaps by stimulating repair processes and activating the body's defenses against further injury.[2,3]

For this reason, licorice or DGL was once a standard European treatment for ulcers.[4] Although it has been replaced by synthetic medications, there is a significant amount of evidence that DGL can be helpful.

DGL is also used for heartburn (esophageal reflux), but we don't know if it simply relieves symptoms or actually protects the esophagus from damage. Licorice (primarily DGL) is also used to relieve the discomfort of canker sores and other mouth sores, based on its mucous membrane–healing capacity.

Creams containing whole licorice (often combined with chamomile extract) are often used for eczema, psoriasis, and herpes.

Whole licorice, not DGL, is used as an expectorant for respiratory problems such as coughs and asthma.

Recently, licorice has been suggested as a treatment for chronic fatigue syndrome (CFS), based on the observation that people with CFS appear to suffer from low levels of certain adrenal hormones. The glycyrrhizin portion of licorice may relieve symptoms by mimicking the effects of these hormones. However, this is a fairly dangerous approach to treatment that should be tried only under medical supervision.

What Is the Scientific Evidence for Licorice?

Several controlled, but not double-blind, studies suggest that regular use of DGL can heal ulcers as effectively as drugs in the Zantac family.[5,6,7] However, DGL must be taken continuously or the ulcer can be expected to return. Modern medical treatment tries to prevent the recurrence of ulcers permanently by eradicating the bacteria *Helicobacter pylori*. There is no evidence that DGL can do the same.

There is no solid evidence for the other proposed uses of licorice.

Dosage

For supportive treatment of ulcer pain along with conventional medical care, chew two to three 380-mg tablets of DGL before meals and at bedtime.

Sucking on these tablets can substantially relieve the discomfort of mouth sores, although some people find the taste unpleasant.

For respiratory problems, take 1 to 2 g of licorice root 3 times daily for no more than 1 week.

For eczema, psoriasis, or herpes, apply licorice cream twice daily to the affected area.

When treating chronic fatigue syndrome, whole licorice must be taken at a sufficiently high dosage so that significant side effects are possible, and thus a physician's supervision is necessary.

Safety Issues

Due to its aldosterone-like effects, whole licorice can cause fluid retention, high blood pressure, and potassium loss when taken at dosages exceeding 3 g daily for more than 6 weeks. These effects can be especially dangerous if you take digitalis, or if you have high blood pressure, heart disease, diabetes, or kidney disease.

DGL is believed to be safe, although extensive safety studies have not been performed. Side effects are rare.

Safety for either form of licorice in young children, pregnant or nursing women, or those with severe liver or kidney disease has not been established.

MAITAKE

(GRIFOLA FRONDOSA)

Principal Proposed Uses

Adaptogen (improve resistance to stress), strengthen immunity

Other Proposed Uses

High cholesterol, high blood pressure, diabetes

Maitake is a medicinal mushroom used in Japan as a general promoter of robust health. Like the similarly described reishi fungus (see Reishi), innumerable healing powers have been attributed to maitake, ranging from curing cancer to preventing heart disease. Unfortunately, there hasn't been enough reliable research yet to determine whether any of these ancient beliefs are really true.

What Is Maitake Used for Today?

Contemporary herbalists classify maitake as an adaptogen, a substance said to help the body adapt to stress and resist infection (see Ginseng for further explanation). However, as for other adaptogens, we lack definitive scientific evidence to show us that maitake really functions in this way.

Most investigation has focused on the polysaccharide constituents of maitake. This family of substances is known to affect the human immune system in complex ways, and one in particular, beta-D-glucan, has been studied for its potential benefit in treating cancer and AIDS.[1,2] Highly preliminary studies also suggest that maitake may be useful in treating diabetes, high blood pressure, and high cholesterol. However, there is no real evidence as yet that maitake is effective for these or any other illnesses.

Dosage

Maitake is an edible mushroom that can be eaten as food or made into tea. A typical dosage of dried maitake in capsule or tablet form is 3 to 7 g daily.

Safety Issues

Maitake is widely believed to be safe, although formal safety studies have not been performed. Safety in young children, pregnant or nursing women, or those with severe liver or kidney disease has not been established.

MARSHMALLOW
(ALTHAEA OFFICINALIS)

Principal Proposed Uses

Cough, asthma, ulcers, diarrhea, Crohn's disease, skin inflammation, sore throat

The similarity in name between the herb marshmallow and the sweet treat is more than a coincidence, although the modern sugar puff ball no longer bears much relationship to the old-fashioned candy flavored with marshmallow herb.

Besides inspiring makers of campfire food, the marshmallow has also been used medicinally since ancient Greece. Hippocrates spoke of it as a treatment for bruises and blood loss, and subsequent Roman physicians recommended marshmallow for toothaches, insect bites, chilblains, and irritated skin. In medieval Europe, herbalists used marshmallow to soothe toothaches, coughs, sore throats, chapped skin, indigestion, and diarrhea.

What Is Marshmallow Used for Today?

Modern herbalists recommend marshmallow primarily for relieving respiratory and digestive problems. The herb contains very high levels of large sugar molecules called mucilage, which appear to exert a soothing effect on mucous membranes. While marshmallow is more a symptomatic treatment than a cure, its ability to soothe a raw throat can be very welcome. It is also sometimes recommended for Crohn's disease or ulcers to reduce discomfort. No double-blind studies have been reported at this time.

Dosage

Marshmallow can be made into a soothing tea by steeping roots overnight in water and diluting to taste. This tea can be drunk as desired for symptomatic relief. Alternatively, you can take marshmallow in capsules (5 to 6 g daily) or in tincture according to label directions.

Marshmallow ointments can be applied directly to soothe inflamed or irritated skin.

Safety Issues

Marshmallow is believed to be entirely safe. It is approved for use in foods, and its chemical makeup does not suggest any but benign effects.[1] However, detailed safety studies have not been performed. One study suggests that marshmallow can slightly lower blood sugar levels.[2] For this reason, people with diabetes should use caution when taking marshmallow. Safety in young children, pregnant or nursing women, or those with severe liver or kidney disease has not been established.

MELISSA a.k.a. LEMON BALM
(MELISSA OFFICINALIS)

Principal Proposed Uses

Topical uses: Oral and genital herpes

Oral uses: Insomnia, nervous stomach

More well known in the United States as lemon balm, *Melissa officinalis* is a native of southern Europe, commonly planted in gardens to attract bees. Its leaves give off a delicate lemon odor when bruised.

Medical authorities of ancient Greece and Rome mentioned topical melissa as a treatment for wounds. The herb was later used orally as a treatment for influenza, insomnia, anxiety, depression, and nervous stomach.

What Is Melissa Used for Today?

Modern German researchers have focused on the ability of melissa creams and ointments to inhibit the herpes virus, as well as the stomach-calming and anti-insomnia benefits of the herb when taken by mouth.

Numerous test-tube studies have found that extracts of melissa possess antiviral properties.[1-4] We don't really know how it works, but the predominant theory is that the herb blocks viruses from attaching to cells.[5]

Melissa cream is used at the first sign of genital or oral herpes. It appears to make flare-ups less intense and last for a shorter period of time, but it doesn't completely eliminate them. There is no evidence that melissa reduces the chances that you can infect someone else. The cream is also applied on a daily basis to prevent flare-ups.

Oral melissa is often used for insomnia and nervous stomach.

What Is the Scientific Evidence for Melissa?

Besides the clinical research described here, see also the description of how melissa cream is made (under Dosage). It, too, provides indirect evidence for melissa's antiviral effect.

Herpes

Early studies of melissa ointments showed a significant reduction in the duration and severity of herpes symptoms (both genital and oral) and, when the cream was used regularly, a marked reduction in the frequency of recurrences.[6,7] In one study, the melissa-treated participants recovered in 5 days, while participants receiving nonspecific creams required 10 days.[8] Researchers also described a "tremendous reduction" in the frequency of recurrence. However, because these studies weren't double-blind, the results can't be taken as reliable.

A subsequent double-blind study followed 116 individuals at two dermatology centers.[9] Treated subjects recovered somewhat more rapidly than those on placebo, although the differences in healing time and size and appearance of lesions weren't huge. People with oral herpes showed a somewhat more marked response than that of those with genital herpes.

To put these findings into perspective, I should note that standard drugs for herpes, such as Zovirax, aren't super-powerful either. In fact, some studies have been unable to show any measurable benefit.[10,11] Zovirax probably does work, but its effects may not be more powerful than those of melissa.

Insomnia

Melissa extracts have also been found to produce a sedative effect in mice.[12] The benefits of combined melissa/valerian extracts in insomnia have been evaluated in one controlled study, discussed under Valerian.[13]

Dosage

For treatment of an active flare-up of herpes, the proper dosage is four thick applications daily of a standardized melissa (70:1) cream. The dosage may be reduced to twice daily for preventive purposes.

The best melissa extracts are standardized by their capacity to inhibit the growth of herpes virus in a petri dish.[14] To make sure the extract has been properly prepared, manufacturers place cells in such a growing medium, and then add herpes virus. Normally, the virus will gradually destroy all the cells. But when little disks containing melissa are added, cells in the immediate vicinity are protected. Although manufacturers use this method to as a form of quality control, it also provides evidence that melissa really works.

When taken orally for its calming effect, the standard dosage of melissa is 1.5 to 4.5 g of dried herb daily.

Safety Issues

Topical melissa is not associated with any significant side effects, although allergic reactions are always possible. Oral melissa is on the FDA's GRAS (generally regarded as safe) list. There are no known drug interactions.

MILK THISTLE

(SILYBUM MARIANUM)

Principal Proposed Uses

Chronic viral hepatitis, acute viral hepatitis, alcoholic liver disease, liver cirrhosis, mushroom poisoning (special intravenous form only)

Milk thistle, a spiny-leafed plant with reddish-purple, thistle-shaped flowers, has a long history of use both as a food and a medicine. English gardeners at the turn of the century grew milk thistle and used the leaves like lettuce, the stalks like asparagus, the roasted seeds like coffee, and the roots (soaked overnight) like oyster plant.

The seeds, fruit, and leaves of milk thistle are used for medicinal purposes. Over 2,000 years ago, Pliny the Elder reported that the juice of milk thistle could "carry off bile," an insight that foreshadowed its modern uses. In Europe, the herb was widely used through the early twentieth century for the treatment of jaundice as well as for insufficient breast milk.

What Is Milk Thistle Used for Today?

Based on the extensive folk use of milk thistle in cases of jaundice, European medical researchers began to investigate its medicinal effects. The results led Germany's Commission E to approve an oral extract of milk thistle as a treatment for liver disease in 1986. It is widely used to treat alcoholic hepatitis, alcoholic fatty liver, liver cirrhosis, liver poisoning, and viral hepatitis. Milk thistle is one of the few herbs that have no real equivalent in the world of conventional medicine.

According to reports and some research evidence that we'll review in the next section, treatment produces a modest improvement in symptoms of chronic liver disease, such as nausea, weakness, loss of appetite, fatigue, and pain. Liver enzymes as measured by blood tests frequently improve, and if a liver biopsy is performed, there may be improvements on the cellular level. Some studies have shown a reduction in death rate among those with serious liver disease.

The active ingredients in milk thistle appear to be four substances known collectively as silymarin, of which the most potent is named silibinin.[1] When injected intravenously, silibinin is one of the few known antidotes to poisoning by the deathcap mushroom, *Amanita phalloides*. Animal studies suggest that milk thistle extracts can also protect against many other poisons, from toluene to acetaminophen.[2-8]

Silymarin appears to function by displacing toxins trying to bind to the liver as well as by causing the liver to regenerate more quickly.[9] It may also scavenge free radicals and stabilize liver cell membranes.[10,11]

However, milk thistle is not effective in treating advanced liver cirrhosis, and only the intravenous form can counter mushroom poisoning.

In Europe, milk thistle is often added as extra protection when patients are given medications known to cause liver problems.

Milk thistle is also used in a vague condition known as minor hepatic insufficiency, or "sluggish liver."[12] This term is mostly used by European physicians and American naturopathic practitioners— conventional physicians don't recognize it. Symptoms are supposed to include aching under the ribs, fatigue, unhealthy skin appearance, general malaise, constipation, premenstrual syndrome, chemical sensitivities, and allergies.

What Is the Scientific Evidence for Milk Thistle?

There is considerable evidence from studies in animals that milk thistle can protect the liver from numerous toxins. However, human studies of people suffering from various liver diseases have yielded mixed results.

Deathcap Poisoning

In *Amanita* mushroom poisoning, silibinin appears to dramatically reduce death rates, which are typically from 30 to 50%, down to less than 10%.[13] This mushroom destroys the liver if left untreated. In conditions like this one, it isn't ethical to perform double-blind studies. However, milk thistle seems to be so dramatically effective that its value is not disputed.

Chronic Viral Hepatitis

Preliminary double-blind studies of people with chronic viral hepatitis have found that milk thistle can produce significant improvement in symptoms such as fatigue, reduced appetite and abdominal discomfort, as well as results on blood tests for liver inflammation.[14,15,16]

Acute Viral Hepatitis

While good results have been reported in one study of 57 people with acute viral hepatitis,[17] another study of 151 participants showed no benefit.[18]

Alcoholic Liver Disease

A 1981 double-blind study followed 106 Finnish soldiers with mild alcoholic liver disease. In the treated group, there was a significant improvement in liver function as measured by blood tests and biopsy.[19]

Another study reported similar results.[20] However, a study of 116 participants showed little to no benefit,[21] as did another study of 72 people followed for 15 months.[22]

Liver Cirrhosis

A controlled study followed 170 people with liver cirrhosis for 3 to 6 years. In the treated group, the 4-year survival rate was 58% as compared to only 38% in the placebo group.[23] However, a recently reported 2-year double-blind study of 200 alcoholics with cirrhosis found no benefit.[24]

Dosage

The standard dosage of milk thistle is 200 mg 2 to 3 times a day of an extract standardized to contain 70% silymarin.

There is some evidence that silymarin bound to phosphatidylcholine may be better absorbed.[25,26] This form should be taken at a dosage of 100 to 200 mg twice a day.

Warning: Considering the severe nature of liver disease, a doctor's supervision is essential. Also, do not inject milk thistle preparations that are designed for oral use!

Safety Issues

Milk thistle is believed to be essentially nontoxic. Animal studies have not shown any detrimental effects even when high doses are given over a long period of time.[27]

A 1992 drug-monitoring study of 2,637 people showed a low incidence of side effects, limited primarily to mild gastrointestinal distress.[28] Although safety in pregnant and nursing mothers has not been proved, based on its extensive food use, researchers have felt safe enough to enroll pregnant women in studies.[29]

MULLEIN
(VERBASCUM THAPSUS)

Principal Proposed Uses

Asthma, colds, cough, ear infections, sore throat

Also called "grandmother's flannel" for its thick, soft leaves, mullein is a common wildflower that can grow almost anywhere. It reaches several feet tall and puts up a spike of densely packed tiny yellow flowers. Mullein has served many purposes over the centuries, from making candlewicks to casting out evil spirits, but as medicine it was primarily used to treat diarrhea, respiratory diseases, and hemorrhoids.

What Is Mullein Used for Today?

Contemporary herbalists sometimes recommend hot mullein tea for asthma, colds, coughs, and sore throats. Mullein seldom produces dramatic effects, but its soothing qualities will be appreciated. You can also breathe the steam from a boiling pot of mullein tea.

Like marshmallow, mullein contains a high proportion of mucilage (large sugar molecules that appear to soothe mucous membranes). It also contains saponins that may help loosen mucus.[1] However, there has not been very much scientific investigation into this popular herb. Mullein is said to be most effective when combined with other herbs of similar qualities, such as yerba santa, marshmallow, cherry bark, and elecampane.

Mullein is also often made into an oily eardrop solution to soothe the pain of ear infections.

Dosage

To make mullein tea, add 1 to 2 teaspoons of dried leaves and flowers to 1 cup of boiling water and steep for 10 minutes. Make sure to strain the tea before drinking it because fuzzy bits of the herb can stick in your throat and cause an irritating tickle.

For painful ear infections, you can squeeze several drops of room-temperature mullein oil into the ear canal, so long as you are sure that the eardrum isn't punctured. But don't expect mullein oil to heal an ear infection: It only relieves the symptoms.

Safety Issues

Mullein leaves and flowers are on the FDA's GRAS (generally regarded as safe) list. Side effects are rare. Nonetheless, safety in young children, pregnant or nursing women, or those with severe liver or kidney disease has not been established.

NEEM

(AZADIRACHTA INDICA)

Principal Proposed Uses

Fevers, respiratory diseases, skin diseases, and other conditions too numerous to list

The neem tree has been called "the village pharmacy," because its bark, leaves, sap, fruit, seeds, and twigs have so many diverse uses in the traditional medicine of India. This member of the mahogany family has been used medicinally for at least 4,000 years, and is held in such esteem that Indian poets called it *Sarva Roga Nivarini*: The One That Can Cure All Ailments. Mohandas Gandhi encouraged scientific investigation of the neem tree as part of his program to revitalize Indian traditions, eventually leading to over 2,000 research papers and intense commercial interest.

At least 50 patents have been filed on neem, and neem-based products are licensed in the United States for control of insects in food and ornamental crops. However, the Indian government and many nongovernmental organizations have united to overthrow some patents of this type, which they regard as "folk-wisdom piracy." One fear is that if neem is patented, indigenous people who already use it will lose the right to continue to do so. Another point is the fundamental question: Who owns the genetic diversity of plants: the nations where the plants come from or the transnational corporations that pay for the research into those plants? Although this area of international law is rapidly evolving, a patent on the spice turmeric has already been overturned, and neem may follow soon.

At least 100 bioactive substances have been found in neem, including nimbidin, azadiracthins, and other triterpenoids and limonoids. Although the scientific evidence for all of neem's uses in health care remains preliminary, the intense interest in the plant will eventually lead to proper double-blind clinical trials.

What Is Neem Used for Today?

The uses of neem are remarkably diverse. In India, the sap is used for treating fevers, general debilitation, digestive disturbances, and skin diseases; the bark gum for respiratory diseases and other infections; the leaves for digestive problems, intestinal parasites, and viral infections; the fruit for debilitation, malaria, skin diseases, and intestinal parasites; and the seed and kernel oil for diabetes, fevers, fungal infections, bacterial infections, inflammatory diseases, and fertility prevention, and as an insecticide.[1,2] Which, if any, of these uses will be verified when proper research is performed remains unclear.

Dosage

Because of the numerous parts of the neem tree used, and the many different ways these can be prepared, the only advice I can give at this time is to follow the directions on the label of the neem product you purchase.

Safety Issues

Based on its extensive traditional use, neem seems to be quite safe. This is particularly remarkable considering that the oil of neem is a powerful insecticide! However, there has not yet been a full scientific evaluation of the toxicity and side effects of neem and its many constituents. At the present time, it is not recommended for use by young children, pregnant or nursing women, or those with severe liver or kidney disease.

NETTLE

(URTICA DIOICA)

Principal Proposed Uses

Benign prostatic hyperplasia (nettle root), allergies (nettle leaf)

Anyone who lives in a locale where nettle grows wild will eventually discover the powers of this dark-green plant. Depending on the species, the fine hairs on its leaves and stem cause burning pain that lasts from hours to weeks. But this well-protected herb can also serve as medicine. Nettle juice was used in Hippocrates' time to treat bites and stings, and European herbalists recommended nettle tea for lung disorders. Nettle tea was used by Native Americans as an aid in pregnancy, childbirth, and nursing.

What Is Nettle Used for Today?

In Europe, nettle root is widely used for the treatment of benign prostatic hyperplasia (BPH), or prostate enlargement. Like saw palmetto, pygeum, and beta-sitosterols, nettle appears to reduce obstruction to urinary flow and decrease the need for nighttime urination. However, the evidence is not as strong for nettle as it is for these other treatments. (For more information on nettle and its use for prostate problems, see *The Natural Pharmacist Guide to Saw Palmetto and the Prostate.*)

Note: Before self-treating with nettle, be sure to get a proper medical evaluation to rule out prostate cancer.

Nettle leaf has recently become a popular treatment for hay fever based on one preliminary study at the National College of Naturopathic Medicine in Portland.

Nettle leaf is also highly nutritious, and in cooked form may be used as a general dietary supplement.

What Is the Scientific Evidence for Nettle?

The evidence is much better for nettle root and prostatic enlargement than for nettle leaf and allergies.

Nettle Root

The use of nettle root for treating benign prostatic hyperplasia has not been as well studied as saw palmetto, but the evidence is at least moderately convincing.

Nettle root contains numerous biologically active chemicals that may influence the function of the prostate, interact with sex hormones, and reduce inflammation.[1-4] Open studies involving a total of over 2,000 men have found significant improvements in prostate size, nighttime urination, urination frequency, urine flow, and residual urine.[5] However, open studies are not necessarily reliable in this case because up to 60% of men with BPH show good responses to placebo.

In a 4- to 6-week double-blind study of 67 men, treatment with nettle produced a 14% improvement in urine flow and a 53% decrease in residual urine.[6] Another double-blind study of 40 men found a significant decrease in frequency of urination after 6 months.[7] A double-blind study of 50 men over 9 weeks found a significant improvement in urination volume.[8]

Nettle Leaf

A preliminary double-blind study suggests that freeze-dried nettle leaf may reduce allergy symptoms.[9]

Dosage

According to Commission E, the proper dosage of nettle root is 4 to 6 g daily of the whole root, or a proportional dose of concentrated extract.

For allergies, the proper dosage is 300 mg twice a day of freeze-dried nettle leaf.

Safety Issues

Because nettle leaf has a long history of food use, it is believed to be safe.

Nettle root does not have as extensive a history to go by. Although detailed safety studies have not been reported, no significant adverse effects have been noted in Germany where nettle root is widely used. In practice, it is nearly side-effect free. In one study of 4,087 people who took 600 to 1,200 mg of nettle root daily for 6 months, less than 1% reported mild gastrointestinal distress and only 0.19% experienced allergic reactions (skin rash).[10]

For theoretical reasons, there are some concerns that nettle may interact with diabetes, blood pressure, and sedative medications, although there are no reports of any problems occurring in real life.

The safety of nettle root or leaf for pregnant or nursing mothers has not been established. However nettle leaf tea is a traditional drink for pregnant and nursing women.

OSHA

(LIGUSTICUM PORTERI)

Principal Proposed Uses

Coughs, respiratory infections, digestive disorders

Native to high altitudes in the Southwest and Rocky Mountain states, the root of the osha plant is a traditional

Native American remedy for respiratory infections and digestive problems. A related plant, *Ligusticum wallichii,* has a long history of use in Chinese medicine, and most of the scientific studies on osha were actually performed on this species.

What Is Osha Used for Today?

Osha is frequently recommended for use at the first sign of a respiratory infection. Like a sauna, it will typically induce sweating, and according to folk wisdom this may help avert the development of a full-blown cold. Osha is also taken during respiratory infections as a cough suppressant and expectorant, hence the common name "Colorado cough root."

Although there have not been any double-blind studies to verify these proposed uses, Chinese research suggests that *Ligusticum wallichii* can relax smooth muscle tissue (perhaps thereby moderating the cough reflex) and inhibit the growth of various bacteria.[1] Whether these findings apply to osha as well is unknown.

Like other bitter herbs, osha also tends to improve symptoms of indigestion and increase appetite.

Dosage

Osha products vary in their concentration and should be taken according to directions on the label.

Safety Issues

Osha is believed to be safe, although the scientific record is far from complete. Traditionally, it is not recommended for use in pregnancy. Safety in young children, nursing women, or those with severe liver or kidney disease has also not been established.

One potential risk with osha is contamination with hemlock parsley, a deadly plant with a similar appearance.[2]

PASSIONFLOWER

(PASSIFLORA INCARNATA)

Principal Proposed Uses

Anxiety, insomnia, nervous stomach

The passionflower vine is a native of the Western hemisphere, named for symbolic connections drawn between its appearance and the crucifixion of Jesus. Native North Americans used passionflower primarily as a mild sedative. It quickly caught on as a folk remedy in Europe and was thereafter adopted by professional herbalists as a sedative and digestive aid.

What Is Passionflower Used for Today?

In 1985, Germany's Commission E officially approved passionflower as a treatment for "nervous unrest." The herb is considered to be a mildly effective treatment for anxiety and insomnia, less potent than kava and valerian, but nonetheless useful. Like lemon balm, chamomile, and valerian, it is also used for nervous stomach.

Animal studies suggest that passionflower extracts can reduce agitation and prolong sleep. There have been no controlled double-blind studies of passionflower in humans, except in combination with other herbs.[1]

Several constituents of passionflower have been credited with causing its sedative effect. However, each has been proven ineffective when used alone. At the current state of knowledge, the best we can say is that we don't yet know how the herb works.

Dosage

The proper dosage of passionflower is 1 cup 3 times daily of a tea made by steeping 1 teaspoon of dried leaves for 10 to 15 minutes. Passionflower tinctures and powdered extracts should be taken according to the label instructions.

Safety Issues

Passionflower is on the FDA's GRAS (generally regarded as safe) list. Although the alkaloids harman and harmaline found in passionflower may increase the effects of drugs known as MAO inhibitors and also stimulate the uterus,[2] it seems unlikely that the normal use of passionflower produces the same effects.

Safety has not been established for pregnant or nursing mothers, very young children, or those with severe liver or kidney disease.

PEPPERMINT

(MENTHA PIPERITA)

Principal Proposed Uses

Irritable bowel syndrome, coughs, colds

Peppermint is a relative of numerous wild mint plants, deliberately bred in the late 1600s in England to become the delightful tasting plant so well known today. It is widely used as a beverage tea and as a flavoring or scent in a wide variety of products.

Peppermint tea also has a long history of medicinal use, primarily as a digestive aid and for the symptomatic treatment of cough, colds, and fever. Peppermint oil is used for chest congestion (Vicks VapoRub), as a local anesthetic (Solarcaine, Ben-Gay), and most recently in the treatment of irritable bowel disease, also known as spastic colon.

What Is Peppermint Used for Today?

Germany's Commission E authorizes the use of peppermint oil for treating colicky pain in the digestive tract (irritable bowel), as well as for relieving mucus congestion of the lungs and sinuses.

What Is the Scientific Evidence for Peppermint Oil?

The scientific record for peppermint oil in treating irritable bowel syndrome is contradictory.

Menthol is the primary ingredient in peppermint oil. Studies have found that it relaxes the muscles of the small intestine in dilutions as low as 1:20,000 and counters the effect of other drugs that cause intestinal spasm.[1,2,3]

Two preliminary double-blind studies, involving a total of 45 individuals with irritable bowel syndrome, found that peppermint can provide significant relief from crampy abdominal pain.[4,5] However, other studies, involving a total of more than 90 people, have found no significant improvement in symptoms.[6,7,8]

The most probable reason for these contradictory results is that peppermint oil is not terrifically effective. Also, the placebo effect is fairly strong in irritable bowel syndrome, making it hard to detect small improvements due to the actual effects of a medicine.

Dosage

The proper dosage of peppermint oil when treating irritable bowel syndrome is 0.2 to 0.4 ml 3 times a day of an enteric-coated capsule. The capsule has to be enteric-coated to prevent stomach distress.

Safety Issues

At the normal dosage, enteric-coated peppermint oil is believed to be reasonably safe in healthy adults.[9,10]

However, if you take too much, peppermint oil can be toxic, causing kidney failure and even death. Excessive intake of peppermint oil can also cause nausea, loss of appetite, heart problems, loss of balance, and other nervous system problems.

Safety in young children, pregnant or nursing women, or those with severe liver or kidney disease has not been established. In particular, peppermint can cause jaundice in newborn babies, so don't try to use it for colic.

A total of at least 200 people have participated in studies of peppermint oil, without any significant problems other than the usual occasional mild gastrointestinal distress or allergic reactions.[11]

PYGEUM
(PYGEUM AFRICANUS)

Principal Proposed Uses

Benign prostatic hyperplasia (prostate enlargement)

Other Proposed Uses

Prostatitis (prostate infection), male impotence, infertility

---

The pygeum tree (pronounced pie-jee-um) is a tall evergreen native to central and southern Africa. Its bark has been used since ancient times to treat problems with urination.

What Is Pygeum Used for Today?

Today, pygeum is primarily used as a treatment for benign prostatic hyperplasia (BPH), or prostrate enlargement, for which purpose it appears to be almost but not quite as effective as saw palmetto. It is more popular in France and Italy than in Germany.

However, saw palmetto is probably the better treatment to use. More is known about it, and furthermore the pygeum tree has been so devastated by collection for use in medicine that some regard it as a threatened species. Saw palmetto is cultivated rather than collected in the wild.

Like other herbs used for prostate problems, pygeum contains many active constituents that are believed to interact with hormones and also inhibit inflammation.[1]

Pygeum is also sometimes used to treat prostatitis, as well as impotence and male infertility.

Note: Before self-treating with pygeum, be sure to get a proper medical evaluation to rule out prostate cancer. (For more information on pygeum, see *The Natural Pharmacist Guide to Saw Palmetto and the Prostate.*)

What Is the Scientific Evidence for Pygeum?

At least nine double-blind trials of pygeum have been performed, involving a total of over 600 people, and ranging in length from 45 to 90 days.[2] Overall, the results make a reasonably strong case that pygeum can reduce such symptoms as nighttime urination, urinary frequency and residual urine volume.

However, a comparison study with saw palmetto found that saw palmetto was more effective than pygeum.[3]

Dosage

The proper dosage of pygeum is 50 to 100 mg twice a day of an extract standardized to contain 14% triterpenes and

0.5 percent n-docosanol. It is often sold at a lower dosage in combination with saw palmetto.

Safety Issues

Pygeum appears to be essentially nontoxic, both in the short and long term.[4] The most common side effect is mild gastrointestinal distress. However, safety in young children, pregnant or nursing women, or those with severe liver or kidney disease has not been established.

RED CLOVER
(TRIFOLIUM PRATENSE)

Principal Proposed Uses
Menopausal symptoms

Other Proposed Uses
Eczema, acne, psoriasis, cancer?

Red clover has been cultivated since ancient times, primarily to provide a favorite grazing food for animals. But, like many other herbs, red clover was also a valued medicine. Although it has been used for many purposes worldwide, the one condition most consistently associated with red clover is cancer. Chinese physicians and Russian folk healers also used it to treat respiratory problems.

In the nineteenth century, red clover became popular among herbalists as an "alterative" or "blood purifier." This medical term, long since defunct, refers to an ancient belief that toxins in the blood are the root cause of many illnesses. Cancer, eczema, and the eruptions of venereal disease were all seen as manifestations of toxic buildup.

Red clover was considered one of the best herbs to "purify" the blood. For this reason, it is included in many of the famous treatments for cancer, including the Hoxsey cancer cure (see Burdock) and Jason Winter's cancer-cure tea. (For more information on cancer prevention, see *The Natural Pharmacist Guide to Reducing Cancer Risk.*)

What Is Red Clover Used for Today?

Recently, an Australian product made from red clover has been marketed as a treatment for menopausal symptoms. It contains high concentrations of four major estrogen-like substances called isoflavones. Studies not yet published at the time of this writing have reportedly found good results. (For more information on menopause and isoflavones, see *The Natural Pharmacist Guide to Menopause.*)

There is no evidence that red clover can help cancer. However, its usage in many parts of the world as a traditional cancer remedy has prompted scientists to take a close look at the herb. It turns out that the isoflavones in red clover may possess antitumor activity.[1,2] However, such preliminary research does not prove that red clover can treat cancer.

Red clover is sometimes recommended for the treatment of acne, eczema, psoriasis, and other skin diseases.

Dosage

A typical dosage of red clover is 2 to 4 g of dried flowers 3 times per day, until symptoms resolve.

Safety Issues

Red clover is on the FDA's GRAS (generally regarded as safe) list, and is included in many beverage teas. However, detailed safety studies have not been performed. Concentrated extracts of red clover may possess dangers not present in beverage teas made from the raw herb. Because of their estrogen-like constituents, red clover extracts should not be used by pregnant or nursing women, or women who have had breast or uterine cancer. Safety in young children, or those with severe liver or kidney disease also has not been established.

Based on their constituents, red clover extracts may conceivably interfere with hormone treatments.

RED RASPBERRY
(RUBUS IDAEUS)

Principal Proposed Uses

Prevent complications of pregnancy

Herbalists have long believed that raspberry leaf tea taken regularly during pregnancy can prevent complications and make delivery easier. Raspberry has also been used to reduce excessive menstruation and relieve symptoms of diarrhea.

What Is Red Raspberry Used for Today?

Red raspberry tea is still commonly recommended for pregnant women.

An interesting study suggests that red raspberry inhibits uterine contractions during pregnancy but not outside of pregnancy.[1] This naturally leads one to wonder whether raspberry leaf first stabilizes the uterus to prevent miscarriages and then somehow turns around and allows the uterus to relax for delivery. However, this is just speculation at the present time. If you take red raspberry during pregnancy, you are doing so based on long tradition, not on science.

Dosage

To make raspberry leaf tea, pour 1 cup of boiling water over 1 or 2 teaspoons of dried leaf, steep for 10 minutes, and then sweeten to taste. Unlike many medicinal herbs, raspberry leaf actually has a pleasant taste! During pregnancy, drink 2 to 3 cups daily.

Safety Issues

Strangely enough, the safety of red raspberry during pregnancy and nursing has not been established. Yet years of traditional use and the widespread availability of the beverage makes it difficult to get very concerned. Safety in young children or those with severe liver or kidney disease has also not been established.

REISHI
(GANODERMA LUCIDUM)

Principal Proposed Uses

Adaptogen (improve resistance to stress), strengthen immunity, improve mental function, prevent altitude sickness

Other Proposed Uses

Asthma, bronchitis, viral hepatitis, cardiovascular disease, ulcers, cancer?

The tree fungus known as reishi has a long history of use in China and Japan as semi-magical healing herb. More revered than ginseng and, up until recently, more rare, many stories tell of people with severe illnesses journeying immense distances to find it. Presently, reishi is artificially cultivated and widely available in stores that sell herb products.

What Is Reishi Used for Today?

Reishi is marketed as a cure-all, said to prevent and treat cancer, strengthen immunity against infection, restore normal immune function in autoimmune diseases (such as myasthenia gravis), improve symptoms of asthma and bronchitis, overcome viral hepatitis, prevent and treat cardiovascular disease, improve mental function, heal ulcers, and prevent altitude sickness. However, there is no real evidence that reishi is effective for any of these conditions.

Contemporary herbalists regard it as an adaptogen, a substance believed to be capable of helping the body to resist stress of all kinds (see discussion of adaptogens under Ginseng). However, while there has been a great deal of basic scientific research into the chemical constituents of reishi, reliable double-blind studies are lacking.

Dosage

The proper dosage of reishi is 2 to 6 g per day of raw fungus, or an equivalent dosage of concentrated extract, taken with meals. Reishi is often combined with related fungi, such as shiitake, hoelen, or polyporus. Results may develop after about 1 to 2 weeks. It is often taken continually for its presumed overall health benefits.

Safety Issues

Reishi appears to be extremely safe. Occasional side effects include mild digestive upset, dry mouth, and skin rash. Reishi can "thin" the blood slightly, and therefore should not be combined with drugs such as Coumadin (warfarin) or heparin. Safety in young children, pregnant or nursing women, or those with severe liver or kidney disease has not been established.

SAW PALMETTO

(SERENOA REPENS OR SABAL SERRULATA)

Principal Proposed Uses

Benign prostatic hyperplasia (prostate enlargement)

Other Proposed Uses

Prostatitis (prostate infection)

Saw palmetto is a native plant of North America, and although Europeans are its principal consumers, it is still primarily grown in the United States.

The saw palmetto tree grows only about 2 to 4 feet high, with fan-shaped serrated leaves and abundant berries. Native Americans used these berries for the treatment of various urinary problems in men, as well as for women with breast disorders. European and American physicians took up saw palmetto as a treatment for benign prostatic hyperplasia (BPH), but in the United States the herb ultimately fell out of favor, along with all other herbs.

European interest endured, and in the 1960s, French researchers discovered that by concentrating the oils of saw palmetto berry they could maximize the herb's effectiveness.

Saw palmetto contains many biologically active chemicals. Unfortunately, we don't know which ones are the most important. We also don't really know how saw palmetto works, although it appears to interact with various sex hormones.

What Is Saw Palmetto Used for Today?

Saw palmetto oil is an accepted medical treatment for benign prostatic hyperplasia (BPH) in New Zealand,

France, Germany, Austria, Italy, Spain, and other European countries. In some countries it is regarded as the "gold standard" against which new prostate drugs must prove themselves!

Typical symptoms of BPH include difficulty starting urination, weak urinary stream, frequent urination, dribbling after urination, and waking up several times at night to urinate. Research suggests that saw palmetto can markedly improve all these symptoms. Benefits require approximately 4 to 6 weeks of treatment to develop and endure for at least 3 years. It appears that about two-thirds of men respond reasonably well.

Furthermore, while the prostate tends to continue to grow when left untreated,[1] saw palmetto causes a small but definite shrinkage.[2,3] In other words, it isn't just relieving symptoms, but may actually be retarding prostate enlargement. The drug Proscar does this too (and to even a greater extent than saw palmetto) but other standard medications for BPH have no effect on prostate size.

Research tells us that saw palmetto is equally effective to Proscar, but it has one great advantage: It leaves PSA (prostate-specific antigen) levels unchanged. Cancer raises PSA levels, and lab tests that measure PSA are used to screen for prostate cancer. Because Proscar lowers PSA measurements, its use may have the unintended effect of masking prostate cancer. Saw palmetto won't do this. On the other hand, Proscar has been shown to reduce the need for surgery, unlike saw palmetto or any of the other drugs used for BPH.

Note: Before self-treating with saw palmetto, be sure to get a proper medical evaluation to rule out prostate cancer.

Saw palmetto is also widely used to treat chronic prostatitis, but its effectiveness in this regard has not been documented.

(For more information on saw palmetto, see *The Natural Pharmacist Guide to Saw Palmetto and the Prostate*.)

What Is the Scientific Evidence for Saw Palmetto?

The science for the effectiveness of saw palmetto in treating prostate enlargement is quite strong, although it could stand to improve.

At least seven double-blind studies involving a total of about 500 people have compared the benefits of saw palmetto against placebo over a period of 1 to 3 months.[4–10] In these studies, the herb significantly improved urinary flow rate and most other measures of prostate disease.[11] Only one study failed to find any benefit. This is fairly impressive, but it would be nice to have a long-term (6 months to 1 year) study of saw palmetto versus placebo.

A double-blind study followed 1,098 men who received either saw palmetto or the drug Proscar over a period of 6 months (unfortunately, there was no placebo group).[12] The treatments were equally effective, but while Proscar lowered PSA levels and caused a slight worsening of sexual function on average, saw palmetto caused no significant side effects.

A recent study involving 435 men found that the benefits of saw palmetto endure for at least 3 years.[13,14] However, there was no control group in this study, making the results unreliable.

Dosage

The standard dosage of saw palmetto is 160 mg twice a day of an extract standardized to contain 85 to 95% fatty acids and sterols. A single daily dose of 320 mg seems to be just as effective.[15] However, taking more than this amount does not seem to produce better results.[16]

Safety Issues

Saw palmetto appears to be essentially nontoxic.[17] It is also nearly side-effect free. In a 3-year study only 34 of the 435 participants complained of side effects—primarily the usual mild gastrointestinal distress.[18] There are no known drug interactions.

Safety for those with severe kidney or liver disease has not been established.

SITOSTEROL

(FROM HYPOXIS ROOPERI)

Principal Proposed Uses

Benign prostatic hyperplasia (prostate enlargement)

Other Proposed Uses

General health benefits

The South African plant *Hypoxis rooperi* has a long history of native use for treating bladder and prostate problems. Its tubers contain a family of cholesterol-like compounds called beta-sitosterols, of which the most important is believed to be beta-sitosterolin. It binds to prostate tissue and affects the metabolism of prostaglandins, substances found in the body that affect pain and inflammation.[1] However, it is not clear whether this is the correct explanation of how sitosterol works or merely an interesting finding.

What Is Sitosterol Used for Today?

For some reason, there seem to be more useful herbal treatments for benign prostatic hyperplasia (BPH), or prostate enlargement, than any other disease (except perhaps varicose veins)! Sitosterol joins saw palmetto, nettles, and pygeum as a documented treatment for BPH.

Based on preliminary evidence, it has been suggested that sitosterols may also offer general health benefits, in particular strengthening the immune system.[2] Sitosterols may eventually take their place alongside flavonoids and carotenes as beneficial substances found in food that aren't essential for life but may enhance overall health. However, more research needs to be done.

(For more information on beta-sitosterol, see *The Natural Pharmacist Guide to Saw Palmetto and the Prostate*.)

What Is the Scientific Evidence for Sitosterol?

One well-designed double-blind placebo-controlled study followed 200 men with BPH for a period of 6 months.[3] Those treated with sitosterol showed significant improvement in many symptoms of prostate enlargement. Smaller studies corroborate these results.[4]

Dosage

The daily dosage of sitosterols should supply 60 to 130 mg of beta-sitosterol. Full effects may take 6 months to develop.

Safety Issues

Although detailed safety studies have not been performed, sitosterol is believed to be safe. No significant side effects or drug interactions have been reported.[5]

SKULLCAP

(SCUTELLARIA LATERIFLORA)

Principal Proposed Uses

Anxiety, insomnia, drug and alcohol withdrawal

Native Americans as well as traditional European herbalists used skullcap to induce sleep, relieve nervousness, and moderate the symptoms of epilepsy, rabies, and other diseases related to the nervous system. In other words, skullcap was believed to function as an herbal sedative.

A relative of skullcap, *Scutellaria baicalensis,* is a common Chinese herb. However, the root instead of the above-ground plant is used, and overall effects appear to be far different. The discussion below addresses European skullcap *(Scutellaria lateriflora)* only.

What Is Skullcap Used for Today?

Skullcap is still popular as a sedative. Unfortunately, there has been virtually no scientific investigation of how well the herb really works. In practice, skullcap seems to produce a mild calming effect, generally not as strong as that of the herb kava, but enough to be helpful at times. It appears to take the edge off mild anxiety and make falling asleep easier. Skullcap is also sometimes used to ease drug or alcohol withdrawal.

Dosage

When taken by itself, the usual dosage of skullcap is approximately 1 to 2 g, 3 times a day. However, skullcap is more often taken in combination with other sedative herbs such as valerian, passionflower, hops, and lemon balm. When using an herbal combination, follow the label instructions for dosage. Skullcap is usually not taken long term.

Safety Issues

Not much is known about the safety of skullcap. However, if you take too much, it can cause confusion and stupor.[1] There have been reports of liver damage following consumption of products labeled skullcap; however, since skullcap has been known to be adulterated with germander, an herb toxic to the liver, it may not have been the skullcap that was at fault. Safety in young children, pregnant or nursing women, or those with severe liver or kidney disease has not been established.

SLIPPERY ELM

(ULMUS RUBRA, ULMUS FULVA)

Principal Proposed Uses

Coughs, irritated digestion, hemorrhoids

The dried inner bark of the slippery-elm tree was a favorite of many Native American tribes, and was subsequently adopted by European colonists. Like marshmallow and mullein, slippery elm was used as a treatment for sore throat, coughs, dryness of the lungs, wounds, skin inflammations, and irritations of the digestive tract.[1] It was also made into a kind of porridge to be taken by weaned infants and during convalescence from illness: Various heroes of the Civil War are said to have credited slippery elm with their recovery from war wounds.

What Is Slippery Elm Used for Today?

Slippery elm has not been scientifically studied to any significant extent. It's primarily used today as a cough lozenge, widely available in pharmacies. Based on its soothing properties, slippery elm is also sometimes recommended for treating irritable bowel syndrome, inflammatory bowel disease (such as Crohn's disease and ulcerative colitis), gastritis, esophageal reflux (heartburn), and hemorrhoids.

Dosage

Suck cough lozenges as needed. For digestive disorders, make a porridge of slippery elm sweetened with honey and eat as desired, or take 500 to 1,000 mg of capsulized powder 3 times daily.

Safety Issues

Other than occasional allergic reactions, slippery elm has not been associated with any toxicity. However, its safety has never been formally studied. Safety in young children, pregnant or nursing women, or those with severe liver or kidney disease has not been established.

STEVIA

(STEVIA REBAUDIANA)

Principal Proposed Uses

Sweetener

This member of the *Aster* family has a long history of native use in Paraguay as a sweetener for teas and foods. It contains a substance known as stevioside that is 100 to 300 times sweeter than sugar, but provides no calories.[1]

In the early 1970s, a consortium of Japanese food manufacturers developed stevia extracts for use as a zero-calorie sugar substitute. Subsequently, stevia extracts became a common ingredient in Asian soft drinks, desserts, chewing gum, and many other food products. Extensive Japanese research has found stevia to be extremely safe. However, there have not been enough U.S. studies for the FDA to approve stevia as a sugar substitute. Without identifying it as such, stevia is nonetheless widely used by savvy manufacturers to sweeten commercial beverage teas and other products.

What Is Stevia Used for Today?

Although some people have claimed that stevia can help regulate blood sugar, the evidence for such an effect is negligible. This dietary supplement is primarily useful as a sweetening agent.

Dosage

Stevia is sold as a powder to be added to foods as needed for appropriate sweetening effects. It tastes slightly bitter if placed directly in the mouth, but in liquids this is generally not noticeable, and most people find the taste delightfully unique.

Safety Issues

Neither animal tests nor the extensive Japanese experience with stevia have uncovered any significant adverse effects.[2,3] However, safety in young children, pregnant or nursing women, or those with severe liver or kidney disease has not been established.

ST. JOHN'S WORT
(HYPERICUM PERFORATUM)

Principal Proposed Uses
Mild to moderate depression

Other Proposed Uses
Anxiety associated with depression, insomnia associated with depression, seasonal affective disorder (SAD)

Probably Ineffective Uses
Viral diseases

St. John's wort is a common perennial herb of many branches and bright yellow flowers that grows wild in much of the world. Its name derives from the herb's tendency to flower around the feast of St. John. (A "wort" is simply a plant in Old English.) The species name *perforatum* derives from the watermarking of translucent dots that can be seen when the leaf is held up to the sun.

St. John's wort has a long history of use in treating emotional disorders. During the Middle Ages, St. John's wort was popular for "casting out demons," conceivably an archaic description of curing mental illness. In the 1800s, the herb was classified as a "nervine," or a treatment for "nervous disorders." It began to be considered a treatment for depression in the early 1900s, and when pharmaceutical antidepressants were invented, German researchers began to look for similar properties in St. John's wort.

Today, St. John's wort is one of the best-documented herbal treatments, with a scientific record approaching that of many prescription drugs. Indeed, this herb *is* a prescription antidepressant in Germany, covered by the national health-care system, and is prescribed more frequently for depression than any synthetic drug.

The active components in St. John's wort are found in the buds, flowers, and newest leaves. Extracts are usually standardized to the substance hypericin, which has led to the widespread misconception that hypericin is the active ingredient. However, there is no evidence that hypericin itself is an antidepressant. Recent attention has focused on another ingredient of St. John's wort named hyperforin as the potential active ingredient. Further research is necessary to confirm this suggestion.

We don't really know how St. John's wort works. Early research suggested that St. John's wort works like the oldest class of antidepressants, the MAO inhibitors.[1] However, later research essentially discredited this idea.[2,3] More recent research suggests that St. John's wort may raise levels of serotonin, norepinephrine, and dopamine. [4,5]

What Is St. John's Wort Used for Today?

St. John's wort is primarily used to treat mild to moderate depression. Typical symptoms include depressed mood, lack of energy, sleep problems, anxiety, appetite disturbance, difficulty concentrating, and poor stress tolerance. Irritability can also be a sign of depression.

Research suggests that St. John's wort is effective in about 55% of cases. As with other antidepressants, the full effect takes approximately 4 to 6 weeks to develop. Although St. John's wort appears to be somewhat less powerful than standard antidepressants, it has one great advantage: It scarcely, if ever, causes side effects.

However, St. John's wort should never be relied on for the treatment of severe depression. If you or a loved one are feeling suicidal, unable to cope with daily life, paralyzed by anxiety, incapable of getting out of bed, unable to sleep, or uninterested in eating, see a physician at once. Drug therapy may save your life.

Furthermore, various systemic diseases may masquerade as depression, such as hypothyroidism, chronic hepatitis, and anemia. Make sure to find out whether you have an undiagnosed medical illness before treating yourself with St. John's wort.

Like other antidepressants, St. John's wort is also used in the treatment of chronic insomnia and anxiety when they are related to depression. It may be effective in relieving seasonal affective disorder (SAD) as well.

Early reports suggested that St. John's wort might be active against viruses such as HIV, but these haven't panned out because unrealistically high concentrations are required.

What Is the Scientific Evidence for St. John's Wort?

None of the double-blind studies of St. John's wort have been particularly large, but taken together they make a convincing case that the herb is an effective antidepressant. There have been two main kinds of studies: those that compared St. John's wort to placebo, and others that compared it to prescription antidepressants.

St. John's Wort Versus Placebo

Probably the best-designed St.-John's-wort-versus-placebo study was reported in 1993 by the German physician K. D. Hansgen and his colleagues.[6] In this 4-week trial, 72 moderately depressed individuals were randomly assigned to receive either placebo or 300 mg 3 times a day of an extract of St. John's wort standardized to contain 0.3% hypericin.

Participants were evaluated using a set of questions called the Hamilton Depression Index (HAM-D). This scale rates the extent of depression, with higher numbers indicating more serious symptoms. Over 80% of the participants taking St. John's wort improved significantly based on this index, while only 26% of the placebo group responded. Later, 36 additional people were added to the trial, with essentially identical results.

A recent double-blind study examined the effectiveness of a new kind of St. John's wort extract standardized to its content of hyperforin rather than to hypericin.[7] It followed 147 people with mild to moderate depression for a period of 42 days. Participants were given either a placebo or one of two forms of St. John's wort: a low hyperforin product (0.5%) or a high hyperforin product (5%).

The results showed that the St. John's wort containing 5% hyperforin was successful in controlling depression symptoms in about 50% of cases, a better result than placebo. Although identical to the high hyperforin product in every respect other than hyperforin content, the low hyperforin product did not do any better than the placebo. This study provides strong evidence that hyperforin is at least one of the active ingredients in St. John's wort.

There have been over 13 other double-blind placebo-controlled studies as well.[8] A review that evaluated most of the published studies found that nine of them were performed according to adequate scientific standards, involving a total of over 600 participants.[9] The combined results make a compelling case for St. John's wort as an effective antidepressant.

This body of research has been criticized by some authorities who point out that none of the studies exceeded 8 weeks in length. However, as it states in the *Physician's Desk Reference*, Prozac was approved on the basis of studies no longer than 6 weeks. It isn't fair to apply a higher standard to herbs than to drugs.

(For more information on St. John's wort, see *The Natural Pharmacist Guide to St. John's Wort and Depression*.)

St. John's Wort Versus Medications

About 10 trials have compared St. John's wort against old-fashioned but tried-and-true antidepressants such as imipramine, maprotiline, and amitriptyline.[10,11,12] Although these studies found generally equal benefits, the dosages of the drugs used were too low to prove much. Instead of the typical 150 to 250 mg a day, participants were only given 50 to 75 mg of the drugs. At these dosages, the drugs didn't really stand a chance of working.

One recent study did use a realistic dose of the drug imipramine, and compared it against double the usual dose of St. John's wort.[13] Interestingly, it followed 209 individuals whose depression was severe rather than mild to moderate. According to the study authors, the results showed that St. John's wort at a double dose was almost as effective as imipramine. However, this seems to be an incorrect reading of the results. St. John's wort was less effective than imipramine, and its performance was not much better than what is usually seen with a placebo. St. John's wort, even at double strength, is probably not an effective treatment for severe depression.

Depression-Related Symptoms

In many of the studies described above, anxiety and insomnia associated with depression were noted to improve with St. John's wort treatment.

Seasonal Affective Disorder

One small, controlled study found St. John's wort to be effective in the treatment of seasonal affective disorder (SAD), a form of depression that occurs primarily during the winter.[14]

Dosage

The standard dosage of St. John's wort is 300 mg 3 times a day of an extract standardized to contain 0.3% hypericin.

A few new products on the market are standardized to hyperforin content (usually 3 to 5%) instead of hypericin. These are taken at the same dosage.

Some people take 500 mg twice a day, or 600 mg in the morning and 300 mg in the evening. If the herb bothers your stomach, take it with food.

Remember that the full effect takes 4 weeks to develop. Don't give up too soon!

Safety Issues

St. John's wort is essentially side-effect free. Strangely, this good news has an unfortunate consequence: Some people who try St. John's wort decide that it must not be very powerful since it doesn't make them feel ill, and quit. Be patient! When St. John's wort works, it is very smooth.

In a study designed to look for side effects, 3,250 people took St. John's wort for 4 weeks.[15] Overall, about 2.4% experienced side effects. The most common were mild stomach discomfort (0.6%), allergic reactions—primarily rash—(0.5%), tiredness (0.4%), and restlessness (0.3%).

In the extensive German experience with St. John's wort as a treatment for depression, there have been no published reports of serious adverse consequences or drug interactions.[16] Animal studies involving enormous doses for 26 weeks have not shown any serious effects.[17]

Cows and sheep grazing on St. John's wort have sometimes developed severe and even fatal sensitivity to the sun. However, this has never occurred in humans taking St. John's wort at normal dosages.[18] In one study, highly sun-sensitive people were given twice the normal dose of the herb.[19] The results showed a mild but measurable increase in reaction to ultraviolet radiation. The moral of the story is that if you are especially sensitive to the sun, don't exceed the recommended dose of St. John's wort and continue to take your usual precautions against burning.

Older reports suggested that St. John's wort works like the class of drugs known as MAO inhibitors.[20] This led to a number of warnings, including avoiding cheese and decongestants while taking St. John's wort. However, this concern is no longer considered realistic. [21,22]

Certain authorities have warned for some time that combining St. John's wort with drugs in the Prozac family (SSRIs) might raise serotonin too much and cause a number of serious problems. Recently, case reports of such events have begun to trickle in. This is a potentially serious risk. Do not combine St. John's wort with prescription antidepressants except on the specific advice of a physician. Since some antidepressants, such as Prozac, linger in the blood for quite some time, you also need to exercise caution when switching from a drug to St. John's wort. (See Transitioning from Medications to St. John's Wort.)

There has also recently been an informal report of St. John's wort lowering blood levels of theophylline, an asthma medication. Preliminary investigation carried out at the University of Colorado suggests that the hypericin in St. John's wort may increase the activity of an enzyme called cytochrome P-450.[23] Throughout evolution, our bodies have developed over 25 different types of this enzyme in our livers and kidneys to break down many naturally occurring chemicals in our diet. Because these enzymes evolved to metabolize many different kinds of natural chemicals, it just so happens that these enzymes break down modern drugs and chemicals, too. Cytochrome P-450 is one of these enzymes. By increasing P-450 activity, St. John's wort may cause the body to speed the breakdown of various drugs (such as theophylline), thereby decreasing their effectiveness. Before taking St. John's wort, it might be a good idea to ask your doctor if any of your medications would be affected by "cytochrome P-450 CYP 1A1 and 1A2 induction."

Finally, preliminary reports from the University of Colorado suggest that St. John's wort may interfere with the action of the antitumor drugs etoposide (VePesid), teniposide (Vumon), mitoxantrone (Novantrone), and doxorubicin (Adriamycin).[24]

Safety in young children, pregnant or nursing women, or those with severe liver or kidney disease has not been established.

Transitioning from Medications to St. John's Wort

If you are taking a prescription drug for mild to moderate depression, switching to St. John's wort may be a reasonable idea if you would prefer taking an herb. Since no one knows whether it is absolutely safe to combine the herb with medications, the safest approach is to stop taking the drug and allow it wash out of your system before starting St. John's wort. Consult with your doctor on how much time is necessary.

However, if you are taking medication for severe depression, switching over to St. John's wort is *not* a good idea. The herb probably won't work well enough, and you may sink into a dangerous depression.

SUMA

(PFAFFIA PANICULATA)

Principal Proposed Uses

Adaptogen (improve resistance to stress), strengthen immunity, enhance exercise ability

Other Proposed Uses

Chronic fatigue syndrome, menopausal symptoms, ulcer disease, anxiety, menstrual problems, aphrodisiac

---

Suma is a large ground vine native to Central and South America. Sometimes called "Brazilian ginseng," native peoples have long used suma to promote robust health as well as to treat practically all illnesses. They called it *Para Toda*, which means "for all things."[1]

What Is Suma Used for Today?

Suma's ancient reputation has generated worldwide interest. However, there has been little formal scientific investigation at this time.

According to most contemporary herbalists, suma is best understood as an adaptogen, a substance that helps one adapt to stress and fight infection (see definition under Ginseng). Along with other adaptogens, Russian Olympic athletes have used suma in the belief that it will enhance sports performance. In the United States, suma is often recommended as a general strengthener of the body, as well as for the treatment of chronic fatigue syndrome, menopausal symptoms, ulcer disease, anxiety, menstrual problems, and low resistance to illness. The herb also enjoys a considerable reputation as an aphrodisiac.

Dosage

A typical dosage of suma is 500 mg twice daily. It is usually taken for an extended period of time.

Safety Issues

Suma has not been associated with any serious adverse reactions. However, comprehensive safety studies have not been undertaken. Safety in young children, pregnant or nursing women, or those with severe liver or kidney disease has not been established.

TEA TREE

(MELALEUCA ALTERNIFOLIA)

Principal Proposed Uses

Wound healing, acne, body odor, fungal infections of the skin, vaginal infections, gum disease

Captain Cook named this tree, after finding that its aromatic, resinous leaves made a satisfying substitute for proper tea. One hundred and fifty years later, an Australian government chemist named A. R. Penfold studied tea tree leaves and discovered their strong antiseptic properties. Tea tree oil subsequently became a standard treatment in Australia for the prevention and treatment of wound infections. During World War II, the Australian government classified tea tree oil as an essential commodity and exempted producers from military service.

However, tea tree oil fell out of favor when antibiotics became widely available.

What Is Tea Tree Used for Today?

There is little question that tea tree oil is an effective antiseptic, active against many bacteria and fungi.[1] It also possesses a penetrating quality that may make it particularly useful for treating infected wounds. However, it is probably not effective as an oral antibiotic.

Like other topical antibiotics, tea tree oil may help control acne when applied to the skin directly.[2] Preliminary studies also hint that it could be useful for treating vaginal infections and fungal infections of the feet and nails. Australian dentists frequently use tea tree oil mouthwash prior to dental procedures and as a daily preventive against gum disease.

Tea tree oil also appears to possess deodorant properties, probably through suppressing odor-causing bacteria.

Dosage

Tea tree preparations contain various percentages of tea tree oil. For treating acne, the typical strength is 5 to 15%; for fungal infections, 70 to 100% is usually used; and for use as a vaginal douche (with medical supervision), 1 to 40% concentrations have been used. It is usually applied 2 to 3 times daily, until symptoms resolve. However, tea tree oil can be irritating to the skin, so start with low concentrations until you know your tolerance.

The best tea tree products contain oil from the *alternifolia* species of *Melaleuca* only, standardized to contain not more than 10% cineole (an irritant) and at least 30% terpinen-4-ol.

Safety Issues

Like other essential oils, tea tree oil can be toxic if taken orally in excessive doses. Since the maximum safe dosage has not been determined, I recommend using it only topically, where it is believed to be quite safe. However, don't get it in your eye or it will sting badly. Safety in young children, pregnant or nursing women, or those with severe liver or kidney disease has not been established.

TURMERIC
(CURCUMA LONGA)

Principal Proposed Uses
Rheumatoid arthritis, osteoarthritis, digestive problems

Other Proposed Uses
Heart disease prevention, cancer prevention

Turmeric is a widely used tropical herb in the ginger family. Its stalk is used both in food and medicine, yielding the familiar yellow ingredient that colors and adds flavor to curry. In the traditional Indian system of herbal medicine known as Ayurveda, turmeric is believed to strengthen the overall energy of the body, relieve gas, dispel worms, improve digestion, regulate menstruation, dissolve gallstones, and relieve arthritis, among other uses.

Modern interest in turmeric began in 1971 when Indian researchers found evidence that whole turmeric possesses anti-inflammatory properties. Much of this observed activity seems to be due to the presence of a constituent called curcumin.[1] Curcumin is also a powerful antioxidant.[2]

What Is Turmeric Used for Today?

Turmeric's antioxidant abilities make it a good food preservative, provided that the food is already yellow in color! It is also reasonable to suppose that turmeric might provide benefits similar to those of other antioxidants, such as vitamin E, in the prevention of heart disease and cancer. However, this has not been proven.

Based on its anti-inflammatory properties, curcumin is commonly recommended as a natural treatment for arthritis as well. One small and highly preliminary double-blind study suggests that curcumin may be helpful in the treatment of rheumatoid arthritis.[3] It also has been suggested for osteoarthritis.

Unlike anti-inflammatory drugs, curcumin does not appear to cause stomach ulcers. But much more and better evidence will be necessary before curcumin can be described as an effective treatment for arthritis. (For more information on arthritis, see *The Natural Pharmacist Guide to Arthritis.*)

Dosage

For medicinal purposes, turmeric is frequently taken in a form standardized to curcumin content, to provide 400 to 600 mg of curcumin 3 times daily.

Unfortunately, curcumin is not absorbed well by the body.[4] It is often sold in combination with bromelain for the supposed purpose of enhancing absorption. While there is no evidence or even sensible reason to believe that this strategy works, bromelain possesses some anti-inflammatory powers of its own that may add to those of curcumin (see Bromelain).

Safety Issues

Turmeric is on the FDA's GRAS (generally recognized as safe) list, and curcumin, too, is believed to be extremely nontoxic.[5,6] Side effects are rare and are generally limited to the usual mild stomach distress. However, safety in young children, pregnant or nursing women, or those with severe liver or kidney disease has not been established.

UVA URSI a.k.a. BEARBERRY

(ARCTOSTAPHYLOS UVA-URSI)

Principal Proposed Uses

Treatment of urinary tract infection (not recommended for prevention of urinary tract infections)

The uva ursi plant is a low-lying evergreen bush whose berries are a favorite of bears; hence the name "bearberry." However, it is the leaves that are used medicinally.

Uva ursi has a long history of use for treating urinary conditions in both America and Europe. Up until the development of sulfa antibiotics, its principal active component, arbutin, was frequently prescribed as a urinary antiseptic.

Although we don't know for sure how uva ursi works, it appears that the arbutin contained in uva ursi leaves is broken down in the intestine to another chemical, hydroquinone. This chemical is altered a bit by the liver and then sent to the kidneys for excretion.[1] In the bladder, it acts as an antiseptic.

Uva ursi appears to be most effective in an alkaline urine, so taking vitamin C with uva ursi probably hampers its work.[2,3]

What Is Uva Ursi Used for Today?

The European Scientific Cooperative on Phytotherapy recommends uva ursi for "uncomplicated infections of the urinary tract such as cystitis when antibiotic treatment is not considered essential."[4] This herb is most useful for women who can tell when they are just starting to develop a bladder infection and can start treatment early. Once you have a severe bladder infection, uva ursi probably won't work very well.

Warning: The herb is definitely not appropriate for kidney infections. If you develop symptoms such as high fever, chills, nausea, vomiting, diarrhea, or severe back pain, get medical assistance immediately.

Furthermore, because hydroquinone can be toxic (discussed under Safety Issues), it isn't a good idea to take uva ursi for a long period of time.

What Is the Scientific Evidence for Uva Ursi?

The research foundation for uva ursi is surprisingly weak considering the popularity of this herb.[5]

Treatment

No double-blind studies have evaluated the clinical effectiveness of uva ursi. However, two studies have evaluated the antibacterial power of the urine of people given uva ursi, and have found activity against most major bacteria that infect the urinary tract.[6,7] This doesn't prove much, however.

Prevention

One double-blind study followed 57 women for one year. Half were given a standardized dose of uva ursi, while the others received placebo treatment. Over the course of the study, none of the women taking uva ursi developed a bladder infection, while five of the untreated women did.[8] However, most experts do not believe that continuous treatment with uva ursi is a good idea (see Safety Issues).

Dosage

The dosage of uva ursi should be adjusted to provide 400 to 800 mg of arbutin daily.[9,10,11] This dosage should not be exceeded, and if the herb is not successful within a week you should definitely seek medical attention. No more than 2 weeks of treatment with uva ursi is recommended, and it should not be used more than five times a year.

Uva ursi should be taken with meals to minimize gastrointestinal upset. Because uva ursi is most effective in alkaline urine, it should not be combined with vitamin C or cranberry juice. You might try taking it along with calcium carbonate or calcium citrate to alkalinize the urine instead.

Uva ursi is also frequently sold in combination with other herbs believed to treat bladder infections, including cleavers, juniper berry, buchu, and parsley.

Safety Issues

Unfortunately, hydroquinone is a liver toxin, carcinogen, and irritant.[12–15] For this reason uva ursi is not recommended for young children, pregnant or nursing women, or those with severe liver or kidney disease.

However significant problems are rare among individuals using prepared uva ursi products in appropriate doses for a short period of time. Gastrointestinal distress (ranging from mild nausea and diarrhea to vomiting) can occur, especially with prolonged use.

VALERIAN
(VALERIANA OFFICINALIS)

Principal Proposed Uses

Insomnia

Other Proposed Uses

Anxiety

Over 200 plant species belong to the genus *Valeriana,* but the one most commonly used as an herb is *Valeriana officinalis*. The root is used for medicinal purposes.

Galen recommended valerian for insomnia in the second century A.D. From the sixteenth century onward, this herb became popular as a sedative in Europe (and later, the United States). Scientific studies of valerian began in the 1980s, leading to its approval as a sleep aid by Germany's Commission E in 1985.

As for most herbs, we are not exactly sure which ingredients in valerian are most important.[1,2] Early research focused on a group of chemicals known as valepotriates, but they are no longer considered candidates. A constituent called valerenic acid is presently under study, but its role is far from clear.

Our understanding of how valerian functions is similarly incomplete. Several studies suggest that valerian affects GABA, a naturally occurring amino acid that appears to be related to the experience of anxiety. Conventional tranquilizers in the Valium family are known to bind to GABA receptors in the brain, and valerian may work similarly. Studies suggest that it either stimulates GABA receptors[3,4] or increases GABA concentrations.[5] However, these hypotheses have been disputed.[6]

What Is Valerian Used for Today?

Valerian is commonly recommended as a mild treatment for occasional insomnia. It appears to be somewhat more effective than herbs such as hops, skullcap, and passion-flower, but less effective than pharmaceutical sleeping pills such as Ambien.

Interestingly, a recent German herbal text suggests that valerian is most useful when taken over an extended period of time.[7] The authors suggest combining valerian extract with a comprehensive sleep-management program for people with chronic sleeping troubles.

Valerian is used to treat anxiety as well, although there is much more scientific evidence for the herb kava.

(For more information on anxiety, see *The Natural Pharmacist Guide to Kava and Anxiety*.)

What Is the Scientific Evidence for Valerian?

The research basis for valerian is growing. The well-designed 28-day study described below still appears to be little known in the United States.

Insomnia

The best study to date of valerian's effectiveness in treating insomnia involved 121 people followed for 28 days.[8] Half of the participants took 600 mg of an alcohol-based valerian extract 2 hours before bedtime, the other half placebo.

At first, placebo and valerian were running neck and neck. But by the end of the study, the participants treated with valerian were definitely sleeping better.

Although positive, these results are a bit confusing because earlier studies showed immediate effects.[9,10] For example, an early double-blind study followed 128 subjects who had no sleeping problems.[11] On three consecutive nights they took either valerian or placebo. The valerian pills significantly reduced the time needed to fall asleep, without affecting dreams or nighttime waking. It is possible that different subspecies of valerian with differing medicinal effects have been used in the various trials.

Finally, a recent double-blind crossover study of 20 people with insomnia compared the benefits of the sleeping drug Halcion (0.125 mg), against placebo and a combination of valerian and lemon balm.[12] Both valerian and Halcion seemed equally effective, but with so few participants the results can't be taken as a reliable indication that this herbal combination is equally effective to Halcion.

Anxiety

Forty-eight participants were placed under situations of "social stress" in a double-blind study of valerian.[13] Individuals in the treated group reported less anxiety.

Animal Studies

Both valerenic acid and whole valerian have been found to produce calming, sleepiness, and reduced activity in laboratory mice.[14–17] Both substances also help prevent seizures. Since most pharmaceutical tranquilizers also reduce seizures, the latter result can be taken as additional indirect evidence of valerian's tranquilizing powers.

Warning: Do not try to substitute valerian for your antiseizure medication. The herb is not powerful enough.

Dosage

For insomnia, the standard dosage of valerian is 2 to 3 g of dried herb, 270 to 450 mg of an aqueous valerian extract, or 600 mg of an ethanol extract, taken 30 to 60 minutes before bedtime.[18]

According to the study mentioned previously that used this dosage, valerian may require weeks to reach its full effects. The same amount, or a reduced dose, can be taken twice daily for anxiety.

Because of valerian's unpleasant odor, European manufacturers have created odorless valerian products. However, these are not yet widely available in the United States.

Valerian is not recommended for children under 3 years old.

Safety Issues

Valerian is on the FDA's GRAS (generally regarded as safe) list, and is approved for use as a food. In animals, even very high doses have not produced serious effects.[19]

There are some safety concerns about valepotriates, constituents of valerian, because they can cause DNA-altering and other toxic effects. However, valepotriates are unstable and not present to a significant extent in any commercial preparations.[20,21]

Except for the unpleasant odor, valerian generally causes no side effects.[22] A few people experience mild gastrointestinal distress, and there have been rare reports of people developing a paradoxical mild stimulant effect from valerian.

Valerian does not appear to impair driving ability or produce morning drowsiness when it is taken at night.[23,24,25] However, there does appear to be some impairment of attention for a couple of hours after taking valerian.[26] For this reason, it isn't a good idea to drive immediately after taking it.

There have been no reported drug interactions with valerian. A 1995 study found no interaction between alcohol and valerian as measured by concentration, attentiveness, reaction time, and driving performance.[27] However, one Japanese study found that valerian extracts prolong drug-induced sleeping time in mice.[28] Thus, it is possible that valerian could compound the effects of other central-nervous-system depressants.

Safety in young children, pregnant or nursing women, or those with severe liver or kidney disease has not been established.

WHITE WILLOW
(SALIX ALBA)

Principal Proposed Uses

Bursitis, tendinitis, headaches, back pain, osteoarthritis, rheumatoid arthritis

---

White willow has been used as a treatment for pain and fever in China since 500 B.C. In Europe, it was primarily used for altogether different purposes, such as stopping vomiting, removing warts, and suppressing sexual desire(!). However, in 1828, European chemists made a discovery that would bring some of these different uses together. They extracted the substance salicin from white willow, which was soon purified to salicylic acid. Salicylic acid is an effective treatment for pain and fever, but it also is sufficiently irritating to do a good job of burning off warts.

Chemists later modified salicylic acid (this time from the herb meadowsweet) to create acetylsalicylic acid, or aspirin.

What Is White Willow Used for Today?

As interest in natural medicine has grown, many people have begun to turn back to white willow as an alternative to aspirin. It is used for many of the same conditions as asprin, such as bursitis, tendinitis, headaches, osteoarthritis, and rheumatoid arthritis. Interestingly, this herb is reportedly not particularly hard on the stomach. This may be due to the fact that most of the salicylic acid in white willow is present in chemical forms that are only converted to salicylic acid after absorption into the body.[1]

Dosage

White willow bark can be made into tea by boiling 1 to 2 g per cup of water for 10 minutes. Standardized tinctures and dry extracts are also available. They should be taken in a dose to provide 60 to 120 mg of salicin daily.[2]

Safety Issues

Although white willow doesn't appear to upset the stomach as easily as aspirin, based on its chemical constituents it is almost certain that it can cause stomach irritation and even bleeding ulcers if used over the long term. All the other risks of aspirin therapy apply as well. For example, white willow should not be given to children, due to the risk of Reye's syndrome. It should also not be used by people with aspirin allergies, bleeding disorders, ulcers, kidney disease, liver disease, or diabetes, and it may interact adversely with alcohol, "blood thinners," other anti-inflammatories, methotrexate, metoclopramide, phenytoin, probenecid, spironolactone, and valproate.

Safety in pregnant or nursing women, or those with severe liver or kidney disease has not been established.

WILD CHERRY
(PRUNUS SEROTINA)

Principal Proposed Uses
Cough

The bark of the wild cherry tree is a traditional Native American remedy for two seemingly unrelated conditions:

respiratory infections and anxiety. European settlers quickly adopted the herb for similar purposes.

What Is Wild Cherry Used for Today?

Over time, wild cherry has come to be used primarily as a component of cough syrups. It is tempting to connect the two traditional uses of wild cherry by imagining that it functions like codeine to affect both the mind and the cough reflex. However, this is just speculation, as there has been very little scientific evaluation of this herb.

Dosage

Syrups containing wild cherry should be taken as directed.

Safety Issues

Wild cherry is generally regarded as safe when used at recommended dosages. However, since it contains small amounts of cyanide, it should not be taken to excess. It is not recommended for use by young children, pregnant or nursing women, or those with severe liver or kidney disease.

WILD YAM
a.k.a. MEXICAN YAM
(DIOSCOREA SPECIES)

Principal Proposed Uses

None

Incorrect Proposed Uses

Source of women's hormones

Various species of wild yam grow throughout North and Central America and Asia. Traditionally, this herb has been used as a treatment for indigestion, coughs, morning sickness, gallbladder pain, menstrual cramps, joint pain, and nerve pain.[1,2] The main use of wild yam in the United States today, however, is based on a fundamental misconception: that it contains women's hormones such as progesterone and DHEA.

In reality, there is no progesterone, DHEA, or any other hormone in wild yam, nor are there any substances that the body can directly use to make such hormones.

To explain this widespread misunderstanding, I have to go back a number of years. When progesterone was first discovered, it was very expensive to produce. The first methods involved direct extraction of progesterone from cow ovaries, a process that required 50,000 cows to yield 20 mg of purified hormone![3] Other hormones such as estrogen and DHEA were also difficult to manufacture. Although doctors wanted to experiment with prescribing these treatments as medicine, until a simpler production method could be developed, it simply wasn't feasible.

The race to discover a more economical source of hormones was won by a scientist/businessman named Russell Marker. In the 1940s, he perfected a method of synthesizing progesterone from a constituent of wild yams called diosgenin. This process involves several chemical transformations carried out in the laboratory.

Marker focused his attention on two species of yam found in Mexico, *Dioscorea macrostachya* and *Dioscorea barabasco*, the latter of which is richer in diosgenin, while the former is much easier to harvest in the wild. He formed a manufacturing company in Mexico that produced progesterone and DHEA from these raw materials.

Unfortunately, corporate competition and difficult labor conditions eventually forced him to close his plant. But Marker's method of synthesizing progesterone continued to be used, bringing the price down drastically and helping to pave the way for the modern birth control pill. Progesterone continued to be manufactured from wild yam for decades, until a cheaper source of raw material was found in cultivated soybeans.

But neither soybeans nor wild yam contain progesterone. They only contain chemicals that chemists can use as a starting point to manufacture progesterone. Furthermore, the body almost certainly can't turn diosgenin into progesterone, because the synthetic steps used by chemists to do so don't even remotely resemble natural processes.[4] Thus, any product that claims to contain "natural progesterone from wild yam" is misleading.

Nonetheless, some wild yam products do contain progesterone. Am I contradicting myself? Not at all: Manufacturers add synthetic progesterone to these creams. There may be a value to taking progesterone in cream form, but the Mexican yam part of the product is a red herring!

YARROW

(ACHILLEA MILLEFOLIUM)

Principal Proposed Uses

Topical uses: Bleeding

Oral uses: Respiratory infections (prevention)

According to legend, the Greek general Achilles used yarrow to stop the bleeding of his soldiers' wounds during the Trojan War: hence the scientific name *Achillea* and the common names "soldier's wound-wort," "bloodwort," and *"herbe militaire."*

Yarrow has also been used traditionally as treatment for respiratory infections, menstrual pain, and digestive upsets.

What Is Yarrow Used for Today?

Like osha, yarrow tea is commonly taken at the first sign of a cold or flu to bring on sweating and, according to tradition, ward off infection. Crushed yarrow leaves and flower tops are also applied directly as first aid to stop nosebleeds and bleeding from minor wounds. However, there has not been any formal scientific study of how well yarrow works.

Dosage

To make yarrow tea, steep 1 to 2 teaspoons of dried herb per cup of water. Combination products should be taken according to label instructions.

Safety Issues

No clear toxicity has been associated with yarrow.[1] The FDA has expressed concern about a toxic constituent of yarrow known as thujone and permits only thujone-free yarrow extracts for use in beverages. Nonetheless, the common spice sage contains more thujone than yarrow, and the FDA lists sage as generally regarded as safe.

Yarrow seldom produces any side effects other than the occasional allergic reaction. Nonetheless, safety in young children, pregnant or nursing women, or those with severe liver or kidney disease has not been established.

YERBA SANTA

(ERIODICTYON CALIFORNICUM)

Principal Proposed Uses

Oral uses: Respiratory diseases

Topical uses: Rash (e.g., poison ivy)

Yerba santa is a sticky-leafed evergreen that is native to the American Southwest. It was given its name ("holy weed") by Spanish priests impressed with its medicinal properties. The aromatic leaves were boiled to make a tea to treat coughs, colds, asthma, pleurisy, tuberculosis, and pneumonia, and a poultice of the leaves was applied to painful joints.

Unlike most medicinal herbs, yerba santa actually has a pleasant taste. It has been used as a general food flavoring and in cough syrups to disguise the bad taste of other ingredients.

What Is Yerba Santa Used for Today?

Some modern herbalists regard yerba santa as one of the most effective natural treatments for chronic respiratory problems such as bronchitis and asthma. Unfortunately, scientific studies of this herb have not been carried out. About the most that can be said is that one of its constituents, eriodictyol, appears to be a mild expectorant.[1]

Yerba santa is occasionally used topically as a treatment for poison ivy.[2]

Dosage

Yerba santa tea may be made by adding 1 teaspoon of crushed leaves to a cup of boiling water and steeping for half an hour. However, because many of its resinous constituents do not dissolve in water, alcoholic tinctures of yerba santa may be more effective. Such tinctures should be taken according to the directions on the label. Drink 3 cups a day until symptoms subside.

Yerba santa is often combined with the herbs osha and grindelia.

Safety Issues

Yerba santa is on the FDA's GRAS (generally regarded as safe) list for use as a food flavoring. There have been no reports of significant side effects or adverse reactions,[3] except for the inevitable occasional allergic reaction. Nonetheless, safety in young children, pregnant or nursing women, or those with severe liver or kidney disease has not been established.

YOHIMBE

(PAUSINYSTALIA YOHIMBE)

Principal Proposed Uses

Impotence (not recommended)

The bark of the West African yohimbe tree is a traditional aphrodisiac and the source of yohimbine, a prescription drug for impotence.

Yohimbine (the drug) is only modestly effective at best, better than placebo but only successful in about 30 to 45% of the men who use it.[1] However, it seems to work even in men whose impotence is caused by a serious illness such as diabetes.

We don't really know how yohimbine works, but recent thinking suggests that it operates by suppressing parts of the brain that keep sexual arousal under control.[2]

In other words, it takes the brake off, which can be useful when the engine has lost some of its power.

What Is Yohimbe Used for Today?

Like the drug yohimbine, the bark of the yohimbe tree is widely used to treat impotence. Many herbalists report that the herb is more effective than the purified drug, perhaps due to the presence of other unidentified active ingredients. However, there have been no good studies to prove this.

Yohimbe is also sometimes recommended as an antidepressant. However, its effectiveness is unknown and there are much safer herbs for this purpose, such as St. John's wort.

Dosage

Yohimbe bark is best taken in a form standardized to yohimbine content. Most people take a dose that supplies 15 to 30 mg of yohimbine daily. However, higher doses are not necessarily better, and some people respond optimally to 10 or even 5 mg daily. Furthermore, while some people appear to respond immediately to a single dose, for others it takes 2 to 3 weeks of treatment to provide significant benefits.

Because yohimbine is a somewhat dangerous substance (see Safety Issues), I recommend a physician's supervision when taking it.

Safety Issues

Yohimbe should not be used by pregnant or nursing women, or those with kidney, liver, or ulcer disease or high blood pressure. Dosages that provide more than 40 mg a day of yohimbine can cause a severe drop in blood pressure, abdominal pain, fatigue, hallucinations, and paralysis. (Interestingly, lower dosages can cause an increase in blood pressure.) Since 40 mg is not very far above the typical recommended dose, yohimbe has what is known as a *narrow therapeutic index*. This means that there is a relatively small dosing range, below which the herb doesn't work and above which it is toxic.

Even when taken in normal dosages, side effects of dizziness, anxiety, hyperstimulation, and nausea are not uncommon.

Yohimbine may also share some properties of a group of rather dangerous antidepressants called monoamine-oxidase inhibitors (MAOIs).[3] While the MAOI-like effects of yohimbine are believed to be weak and probably not significant, it may be prudent to use typical MAOI precautions, such as avoiding cheese, red wine, liver, and other tyramine-containing foods.

Yohimbe is not recommended for young children, pregnant or nursing women, or those with severe liver or kidney disease.

YUCCA
(YUCCA BREVIFOLIA AND OTHER SPECIES)

Principal Proposed Uses
Arthritis (both rheumatoid and osteoarthritis)

Various species of yucca plant were used as food by Native Americans and early California settlers. Yucca contains high levels of soapy compounds known as saponins that also made it a useful natural shampoo and soap.

What Is Yucca Used for Today?
When taken for a long period of time, yucca is said to reduce arthritis symptoms. However, the only scientific

evidence for this claim comes from one preliminary study.[1] (For more information on arthritis, see *The Natural Pharmacist Guide to Arthritis.*)

Yucca extracts are also widely used to enhance the foaming effect of carbonated beverages.

Dosage

The standard dosage is 2 to 4 tablets of concentrated yucca saponins daily.

Safety Issues

Yucca is generally accepted as safe based on its long history of use as a food. However, it sometimes causes diarrhea if taken to excess. Safety in young children, pregnant or nursing women, or those with severe liver or kidney disease has not been established.

Chinese Herbal Combinations

As described in the introduction, Chinese herbal medicine is quite different from the usual way of using herbs. Rather than using one or more herbs based on particular diseases or symptoms, it relies on complex combinations custom-blended to the particular needs of the individual. This makes Chinese medicine not well suited to self-care.

However, a few standard herbal combinations for common diseases have become popular medicine-chest items in China, and many of these are available in the United States as well. One common name for these formulas is "patent medicine."

This section briefly discusses a few of the most ubiquitous Chinese patent products. Many of these treatments often seem quite effective in practice. However, if you choose to use any, keep in mind the following realities:

- This is not the best way to use Chinese medicine. Many properly qualified herbal practitioners frown on the use of these patent remedies. Formulas are supposed to be individualized.
- Manufacturing standards in China are rather lax. The ingredients of patent remedies may change from year to year, and these changes are not always reflected on the labeling.

- There are concerns that relatively high levels of pesticides and other contaminants (including prescription drugs) may be present in some of these products.
- Besides the risk of contaminants, the safety of the actual herbs used in these formulas has not been extensively investigated.
- Finally, there is no real scientific evidence for the effectiveness of these herbal remedies. Their use is based entirely on Chinese herbal tradition.

Despite these objections, millions of people use herbal formulations such as those described in this section without apparent harm. In no case, however, would I recommend that pregnant or nursing women use these herbs.

BI YAN PIAN
(RHINITIS TABLETS);

PE MIN KAN WAN
(NASAL CLEAR)

Principal Proposed Uses
Nasal and sinus congestion

These are the two most common patent remedies for relieving nasal stuffiness. Bi Yan Pian is generally recommended for actual sinus infections, while Pe Min Kan Wan is more properly used for sinus allergies, but the two are similar enough that they are often used interchangeably.

Ingredients

Bi Yan Pian consists of the following ingredients: *Fructus xanthii* 22.5%, *Flox magnoliae liliforlae* 22.5%, *Radix glycyrrhizae uralensis* 6.5%, *Cortex phellodendri* 6.5%, *Radix platycodi* 4.15%, *Fructus shizandra chinensis* 4.15%, *Fructus forsythiae suspensae* 6.5%, *Radix angelicae* 6.5%, *Rhizoma anemarrhenae ashphodeloidis* 4.15%, *Flos chrysanthemi indicae indici* 4.15%, *Herba ledebouriellae sesloidis* 4.15%, and *Herba seu flos schizonepetae tenuifoliae* 4.15%.[1]

Pe Min Kan Wan's constituents appear to vary from time to time, but a recent product bulletin states that it contains *Radix scutellariae* 26%, *Xanthii fructus* 25%, *Herba centipedae* 14% (a euphemism for centipede!), *Agastaches heba* 25%, and *Angelicae cigantis rhizoma* 10%.[2]

Dosage

Bi Yan Pian is taken at a dosage of 3 to 4 tablets, 3 times daily after meals. It is usually used only for a few weeks. The manufacturer suggests that this dose should not be exceeded due to the "slight toxicity" of *Fructus Xanthiis*.[3] What this term really means, how the manufacturers know that it is toxic, and under what conditions and for whom it may be dangerous remain unclear.

Pe Min Kan Wan is taken at a dosage of 2 to 3 pills, 3 times daily, for up to 4 months.

Safety Issues

In practice, noticeable side effects are rare for these two products. However, as for all Chinese herbal patent formulas, the actual safety of Bi Yan Pian and Pe Min Kan Wan has not been established. Pregnant or nursing women absolutely should not take either of these products.

PO CHAI

(CURING PILLS)

Principal Proposed Uses

Digestive distress

These two nearly identical patent medicines can be found in almost every Chinese medicine chest, and they have become increasingly prevalent in the United States as well. Curing Pills (also known as Pill Curing, and Healthy and Quiet Pills) and Po Chai are used for practically any minor digestive upset, including overeating, indigestion, motion sickness, stomach flu, and alcoholic hangovers. Many people report rapid, dramatic relief. Traditionally, these are short-term remedies only that should not be taken continuously for chronic digestive problems.

Ingredients

Curing Pills consist of *Rhizoma gastrodiae elatae* 3.6%, *Radix angelicae* 7.2%, *Flos chrysanthemi indicae morifolii* 3.7%, *Herba menthae* 3.2%, *Radix puerariae lobetae* 7.2%, *Radix tricosanthis* 5.5%, *Radix atractylodes* 7.2%, *Semen coicis lachryma-jobi* 9%, *Sclerotium poriae cocus* 15.5%, *Radiz saussureae seu vladimiriae* 7.2%, *Cortex magnoliae officinalis* 7.2%, *Pericarpium citri erythrocarpae* 3.6%, *Herba agastaches seu pogostemi* 7.2%, *Mass medica fermentata* 7.2% and *Fructus oryzae sativae germinatis* 5.5%.[1]

The ingredients of Po Chai are not much different.

Dosage

Curing Pills come in little vials, each of which contains many small pellets. The usual dosage is 1 to 2 vials (that's whole vials, not pellets!), up to 3 times a day. The dosage for Po Chai is the same.

Safety Issues

As for all Chinese patent remedies, proper scientific safety testing has not been performed. I certainly wouldn't recommend that pregnant or nursing women take Curing Pills. However, noticeable side effects are rare.

YIN CIAO

(TOXIN-VANQUISHING TABLETS)

Principal Proposed Uses

Flus

Yin Ciao tablets (also written Yin Chiao, and Yin Qiao Jie Du Pian) are yet another staple medicine-cabinet item, used as first aid for flus and other respiratory infections. Technically, this formula is meant to be used in cases of "wind heat," a classic Chinese medical diagnosis that deserves an explanation.

In Chinese medicine, respiratory infections are frequently described as being due to "wind." The average common cold would be classified as "wind cold," with mild fever, a sense of chilliness, a mildly uncomfortable sensation in the muscles, and respiratory symptoms. In contrast, "wind heat" more closely resembles what we would call a flu, with higher fever, severe muscle aches, intense fatigue, and headache.

Yin Ciao is traditionally used for symptomatic relief at the first sign of an obvious flu (not a stomach flu, but a classic ache-all-over attack of influenza). It is not supposed to be used for colds.

Yin Ciao is also used to treat some forms of tonsillitis and other infections, but it takes a qualified herbalist to determine whether a particular infection matches the traditional function of this combination.

However, there is no scientific evidence whatsoever that Yin Ciao is effective. It definitely should *not* be relied upon to treat any potentially serious infections, such as strep throat or severe influenza.

Ingredients

Yin Ciao generally consists of *Flos lonicerae japonicae* 17.76%, *Fructus forsythiae suspensae* 17.76%, *Fructus arctii* 10.6%, *Radix platycodi* 10.66%, *Herba menthae* 10.66%, *Rhizoma phragmatis* 8.88%, *Herba lphatheri* 7.1%, *Raiz glycyrrhizae uralensis* 8.88%, and *Herba ser flos schizonopetae tenuifoliae* 7.10%.[1] However, the ingredients vary from time to time, and some year's products have been known to contain Western drugs such as antihistamines and caffeine.

Dosage

Because there are many forms of Yin Ciao available, it should be taken according to the directions on the label.

Safety Issues

Because Yin Ciao has never been properly studied to evaluate its safety, pregnant or nursing women should not use it. However, noticeable side effects are rare and mostly limited to mild allergic reactions.

Notes

Aloe

1. Marshall HM. *Aloe vera* gel: What is the evidence? *Pharmacol J* 244: 360–362, 1990.

2. Schmidt JM, et al. *Aloe vera* dermal wound gel is associated with a delay in wound healing. *Obstet Gynecol* 78: 115–117, 1991.

3. Hart LA, et al. Effects of low molecular weight constituents from *Aloe vera* gel on oxidative metabolism and cytotoxic and bactericidal activities of human neutrophils. *Int J Immunol Pharmacol* 12: 427–434, 1990.

4. Sheets MA, et al. Studies of the effect of acemannan on retrovirus infections: Clinical stabilization of feline leukemia virus-infected cats. *Mol Biother* 3: 41–45, 1991.

5. Kemp MC, et al. In-vitro evaluation of the antiviral effects of acemannan on the replication and pathogenesis of HIV-1 and other enveloped viruses: Modification of the processing of glycoprotein precursors. *Antiviral Res* 13(Suppl. 1): 83, 1990.

Andrographis

1. Hancke J, et al. A double-blind study with a new monodrug Kan Jang: Decrease of symptoms and improvements in the recovery from common colds. *Phytotherapy Res* 9: 559–562, 1995.

2. Melchior J, et al. Controlled clinical study of standardized *Andrographis paniculata* extract in common cold: A pilot trial. *Phytomedicine* 34: 314–318, 1996–1997.

3. Hancke J, et al. 1995.

4. Thamlikitkul V, et al. Efficacy of *Andrographis paniculata* (Nees) for pharyngotonsillitis in adults. *J Med Assoc Thai* 74(10): 437–442, 1991.

5. Hancke J, et al. 1995.

6. Akbarsha MA, et al. Antifertility effect of *Andrographis paniculata* (Nees) in male albino rat. *Indian J Exp Biol* 28(5): 421–426, 1990.

7. Burgos RA, et al. Testicular toxicity assessment of *Andrographis paniculata* dried extract in rats. *J Ethnopharmacol* 58(3): 219–224, 1997.

8. Zoha MS, et al. Antifertility effect of *Andrographis paniculata* in mice. *Bangladesh Med Res Counc Bull* 15(1): 34–37, 1989.

Ashwaganda

1. Devi PU, et al. In vivo growth inhibitory effect of *Withania somnifera* (ashwaganda) on a transplantable mouse tumour, Sarcoma 180. *Indian J Exp Biol* 30: 169–172, 1992.

2. Al-Hindawi MK, et al. Anti-granuloma activity of Iraqi *Withania somnifera*. *J Ethnopharmacol* 37: 113–116, 1992.

3. Kuppurajan K, et al. Effect of ashwaganda (*Withania somnifera Dunal*) on the process of aging in human volunteers. *J Res Ayurveda Siddha* 1: 247–258, 1980.

4. Bone, K. MediHerb Professional Newsletter No. 30 Warwick, Australia, 1998.

Astragalus

1. Benksy D and Gamble A. Chinese herbal medicine: Materia medica. Seattle, WA: Eastland Press, 1986: 457–459.

2. Hou Y, et al. Effect of *Radix Astragali Seu Hedysari* on the interferon system. *Chin Med J* 94: 35–40, 1981.

3. Sun Y, et al. Immune restoration and/or augmentation of local graft versus host reaction by traditional Chinese medicinal herbs. *Cancer* 52: 70–73, 1983.

4. Benksy D and Gamble A. 1986.

5. Liang R, et al. Clinical study on braincalming tablets in treating 450 cases of atherosclerosis. *J North Chin Med* 1: 63–65, 1985.

6. Xiao S. et al. Hyperthyroidism treated with yiqiyangyin decoction. *J Trad Chin Med* 6(2): 79–82, 1986.

7. Zhang ND, et al. Effects on blood pressure and inflammation of astragalus saponin 1, a principle isolated from *Astragalus membranaceus* Bge. *Acta Pharm Suec* 19(5): 333–337, 1984.

8. Zhang H, et al. Treatment of adult diabetes with jiangtangjia tablets. *J Trad Chin Med* 7(4): 37–39, 1986.

9. Zhou MX, et al. Therapeutic effect of astragalus in treating chronic active hepatitis and the changes in immune function. *J Chin People's Liberation Army* 7(4): 242–244, 1982.

10. Benksy D and Gamble A. 1986.

Bilberry

1. Monboisse JC, et al. Non-enzymatic degradation of acid-soluble calf skin collagen by superoxide ion: Protective effect of flavonoids. *Biochem Pharmacol* 32: 53–58, 1983.

2. Havsteen B. Flavonoids, a class of natural products of high pharmacological potency. *Biochem Pharmacol* 32: 1141–1148, 1983.

3. Gabor M. Pharmacologic effects of flavonoids on blood vessels. *Angiologica* 9: 355–374, 1972.

4. Mian E, et al. Anthocyanosides and the walls of microvessels: Further aspects of the mechanism of action of their protective effect in syndromes due to abnormal capillary fragility. *Minerva Med* 68: 3565–3581, 1977.

5. Puilleiro G, et al. Ex vivo study of the inhibitory effects of *Vaccinium myrtillus* anthocyanosides on human platelet aggregation. *Fitoterapia* 60: 69–75, 1989.

6. Wegmann R, et al. Effects of anthocyanosides on photoreceptors. Cyto-enzymatic aspects. *Ann Histochim* 14: 237–256, 1969.

7. Bone K, et al. Mediherb Professional Review. 59(3): 1997.

8. Bone K, et al. 1997.

9. Sala D, et al. Effect of anthocyanosides on visual performance at low illumination. *Minerva Oftalmol* 21: 283–285, 1979.

10. Gloria E, et al. Effect of anthocyanosides on the absolute visual threshold. *Ann Ottalmol Clin Ocul* 92: 595–607, 1966.

11. Caselli L. Clinical and electroretinographic study on activity of anthocyanosides. *Arch Intern Med* 37: 29–35, 1985.

12. Bone K, et al. 1997.

13. Bone K, et al. 1997.

14. Scharrer A, et al. Anthocyanosides in the treatment of retinopathies. *Klin Monatsbl Augenheilkd* 178: 386–389, 1981.

15. Bravetti G. Preventive medical treatment of senile cataract with vitamin E and anthocyanosides: Clinical evaluation. *Ann Ottalmol Clin Ocul* 115: 109, 1989.

16. Bone K, et al. 1997.

17. Bone K, et al. 1997.

18. Ghiringhelli C, et al. Capillarotropic activity of anthocyanosides in high doses in phlebopathic stasis. *Minerva Cardioangiol* 26: 255–276, 1978.

19. Grismond GL. Treatment of pregnancy-induced phlebopathies. *Minerva Ginecol* 33: 221–230, 1981.

20. Lietti A, et al. Studies on *Vaccinium myrtillus* anthocyanosides. I. Vasoprotective and anti-inflammatory activity. *Arzneimittelforschung* 26: 829–832, 1976.

21. Lietti A, et al. Studies on *Vaccinium myrtillus* anthocyanosides. II. Aspects of anthocyanin pharmacokinetics in the rat. *Arzneimittelforschung* 26: 832–835, 1976.

22. Eandi M. Unpublished results cited in Morazzoni P, et al. *Vaccinium myrtillus*. *Fitoterapia* 67(1): 3–29, 1996.

23. Grismond GL. 1981.

Bitter Melon

1. Srivastava Y, et al. Antidiabetic and adaptogenic properties of *Momordica charantia* extract: An experimental and clinical evaluation. *Phytother Res* 7: 285–289, 1993.

2. Welihinda J, et al. The insulin-releasing activity of the tropical plant *Momordica charantia*. *Acta Biol Med Germ* 41: 1229–1240, 1982.

3. Murray M. The healing power of herbs. Rocklin, CA: Prima Publishing, 1995: 358.

Black Cohosh

1. Jarry H, et al. II. Endocrine effects of constituents of *Cimicifuga racemosa*. 1. The effect on serum levels of pituitary hormones in ovariectomized rats. *Planta Med* 1: 46–49, 1985.

2. Jarry H, et al. The endocrine effects of constituents of *Cimicifuga racemosa*. 2. In vitro binding of constituents to estrogen receptors. *Planta Med* 4: 316–319, 1985.

3. Duker EM, et al. Effects of extracts from *Cimicifuga racemosa* on gonadotropin release in menopausal women and ovariectomized rats. *Planta Med* 57(5): 420–424, 1991.

4. Stolze H. An alternative to treat menopausal complaints. *Gyne* 3: 14–16, 1982.

5. Schulz V, et al. Rational phytotherapy. New York: Springer-Verlag, 1998: 246.

6. Warnecke G. Influencing menopausal symptoms with a phytotherapeutic agent. *Med Welt* 36: 871–874, 1985.

7. Stoll W. Phytopharmacon influences atrophic vaginal epithelium. Double-blind study: Cimicifuga vs. estrogenic substances. *Therapeuticum* 1: 23–31: 1987.

8. Schaper and Brümmer Remifemin®: A plant-based gynecological agent. Scientific brochure, 1997.

9. Jones TK, et al. Profound neonatal congestive heart failure caused by maternal consumption of blue cohosh herbal medication. *J Pediatr* 132: 550–552, 1998.

10. Korn WD. Six-month oral toxicity study with Remifemin-granulate in rats followed by an 8-week recovery period. Hannover, Germany: International Bioresearch, 1991.

11. Nesselhut T, et al. Influence of *Cimicifuga racemosa* extracts with estrogen-like activity on the in vitro proliferation of mammalian carcinoma cells. *Arch Gynecol Obstet* 254: 817–818, 1993.

12. Newall C. Herbal medicines: A guide for health-care professionals. London: Pharmaceutical Press, 1996: 80.

Bloodroot

1. Godowski KC. Antimicrobial action of sanguinarine. *J Clin Dentistry* 1: 96–101, 1989.

2. Lawrence Review of Natural Products. Bloodroot monograph. St. Louis, MO: Facts and Comparisons Division, J. B. Lipincott Company, 1992.

3. Newall C, et al. Herbal medicines: A guide for health-care professionals. London: Pharmaceutical Press, 1996: 42–43.

Boswellia

1. Safyhi H, et al. 5-lipoxygenase inhibition by acetyl-11-keto-b-boswellic acid. *Phytomedicine* 3: 71–72, 1996.

2. Singh G, et al. Pharmacology of an extract of salai guggal ex-*Bosewellia serrata,* a new non-steroidal anti-inflammatory agent. *Agents Action* 18: 407–412, 1986.

3. Reddy CK, et al. Studies on the metabolism of glycosaminoglycans under the influence of new herbal anti-inflammatory agents. *Biochem Pharmacol* 20: 3527–3534, 1989.

4. Etzel R. Special extract of *Boswellia serrata* in the treatment of rheumatoid arthritis. *Phytomed* 3(1): 67–70, 1996.

5. Sander O, Herborn G, and Rau R. Is H15 resin extract of *Boswellia serrata* "incense" a useful supplement to established drug therapy of chronic polyarthritis? Results of a double-blind pilot study (Eng Abst Only). *Z Rheumatol* 57(1): 11–16, 1998.

Bromelain

1. Taussig S, et al. Bromelain, a proteolytic enzyme and its clinical application. A review. *Hiroshima J Med Sci* 24: 185–193, 1975.

2. Taussig S, et al. Bromelain, the enzyme complex of pineapple (*Ananas comosus*) and its clinical application. An update. *J Ethnopharmacol* 22: 191–203, 1988.

3. Schulz V, et al. Rational phytotherapy. New York: Springer-Verlag, 1998: 263.

4. Schulz V, et al. 1998.

5. Izaka K, et al. Gastrointestinal absorption and anti-inflammatory effect of bromelain. *Jpn J Pharmacol* 22: 519–534, 1972.

6. Seligman B. Bromelain: An anti-inflammatory agent. *Angiology* 13: 508–510, 1962.

7. Pirotta F, et al. Bromelain—A deeper pharmacological study. Note I. Anti-inflammatory and serum fibrinolytic activity after oral administration in the rat. *Drugs Exp Clin Res* 4: 1–20, 1978.

8. Schulz V, et al. 1998.

9. Seligman B. 1962.

10. Blonstein J. Control of swelling in boxing injuries. *Practitioner* 203: 206, 1960.

11. Blumenthal M, et al. The complete German Commission E monographs. Boston: Integrative Medicine Communications, 1998: 94.

Burdock

1. Newall C, et al. Herbal medicines: A guide for health-care professionals. London: Pharmaceutical Press, 1996: 52–53.

Butcher's Broom

1. Bouskela E, et al. Effects of Ruscus extract on the internal diameter of arterioles and venules of the hamster cheek pouch microcirculation. *J Cardiovasc Pharmacol* 22: 221–224, 1993.

2. Bouskela E, et al. Inhibitory effect of the Ruscus extract and of the flavonoid heperidine methylchalcone on increase microvascular permeability induced by various agents in the hamster cheek pouch. *J Cardiovasc Pharmacol* 22: 225–230, 1993.

Calendula

1. Schulz V, et al. Rational phytotherapy. New York: Springer-Verlag, 1998: 259.

2. Lawrence Review of Natural Products. Calendula monograph. St. Louis, MO: Facts and Comparisons Division, J. B. Lipincott Company, 1995.

3. Schulz V, et al. 1998.

Cat's Claw

1. Jones K. Cat's claw. *Herbs for Health* September/October: 42–46, 1996.

2. Lininger S, et al. The natural pharmacy. Rocklin, CA: Prima Publishing, 1998: 246.

Cayenne

1. Graham DY, et al. Spicy food and the stomach: Evaluation by videoendoscopy. *JAMA* 260(23): 3473–3475, 1988.

Chamomile

1. Hormann HP, et al. Evidence for the efficacy and safety of topical herbal drugs in dermatology: Part 1. Anti-inflammatory agents. *Phytomedicine* 1: 161–167, 1994.

2. Schulz V, et al. Rational phytotherapy. New York: Springer-Verlag, 1998: 254–256.

3. Schulz V, et al. 1998: 256.

Chasteberry

1. Milewicz A, et al. *Vitex agnus-castus* extract in the treatment of luteal phase defects due to latent hyperprolactinemia. Results of a randomized placebo-controlled double-blind study. *Arzneimittelforschung* 43(7): 752–756, 1993.

2. Jarry H, et al. In vitro prolactin but not LH and FSH release is inhibited by compounds in extracts of *Agnus castus:* Direct evidence for a dopaminergic principle by the dopamine receptor assay. *EYP Clin Endocrinol* 102: 448–454, 1994.

3. Sliutz G, et al. *Agnus castus* extracts inhibit prolactin secretion of rat pituitary cells. *Horm Metab Res* 25(5): 253–255, 1993.

4. Schulz V, et al. Rational phytotherapy. New York: Springer-Verlag, 1998: 241–242.

5. Propping D, et al. Diagnosis and therapy of corpus luteum insufficiency in general practice. *Therapiewoche* 38: 2992–3001, 1988.

6. Dittmar FW, et al. Premenstrual syndrome: Treatment with a phytopharmaceutical. *Therapiewoche Gynakol* 5: 60–68, 1992.

7. Peteres-Welte C, et al. Menstrual abnormalities and PMS: *Vitex agnus-castus. Therapiewoche Gynakol* 7: 49–52, 1994.

8. Lauritzen C, et al. Treatment of premenstrual tension syndrome with *Vitex agnus-castus*. Controlled, double-blind study vs. pyridoxine. *Phytomedicine* 4(3): 183–89, 1997.

9. Lauritzen C, et al. 1997.

10. Kleijnen J, et al. Vitamin B_6 in the treatment of PMS—A review. *Br J Obstet Gynaecol* 97: 847–852, 1990.

11. Milewicz A, et al. 1993.

12. Schulz V, et al. 1998: 243.

13. Cahill DJ, et al. Multiple follicular development associated with herbal medicine. *Hum Reprod* 9(8): 1469–1470, 1994.

Coleus forskohlii

1. Seamon KB and Daly JW. Forskolin: A unique diterpene activator of cAMP-generating systems. *J Cyclic Nucleotide Res* 7: 201–224, 1981.

2. Laurenza A, Sutkowski EM, and Seamon KB. Forskolin: A specific stimulator of adenylyl cyclase or a diterpene with multiple sites of action? *Trends Pharmacol Sci* 10: 442–447, 1989.

3. Marone G, et al. Forskolin inhibits the release of histamine from human basophils and mast cells. *Agents Actions* 18: 96–99, 1986.

4. Ammon HPT, et al. Forskolin: From Ayurvedic remedy to a modern agent. *Planta Med* 51: 473–477, 1985.

5. DeSouza NJ. Industrial development of traditional drugs: The forskolin example. A mini-review. *J Ethnopharmacol* 38: 1177–1180, 1993.

6. Kreutner W, et al. Bronchodilatory and antiallergy activity of forskolin. *Eur J Pharmacol* 11: 1–8, 1985.

7. Schlepper M, et al. Cardiovascular effects of forskolin and phophodiesterase-III inhibitors. *Basic Res Cardiol* 84(Suppl. 1): 197–212, 1989.

8. Dubey MP, et al. Pharmacological studies on coleonol, a hypotensive diterpene from *Coleus forskohlii*. *J Ethnopharmacol* 3: 1–13, 1981.

9. Bauer K, et al. Pharmacodynamic effects of inhaled dry powder formulations of fenoterol and colforsin in asthma. *Clin Pharmacol Ther* 53: 76–83, 1993.

10. Meyer BH, et al. The effects of forskolin eye drops on intraocular pressure. *S Afr Med J* 71(9): 570–571, 1987.

Cranberry

1. Sobota AE. Inhibition of bacterial adherence by cranberry juice: Potential use for the treatment of urinary tract infections. *J Urol* 131: 1013–1016, 1984.

2. Schmidt DR, et al. An examination of the anti-adherence activity of cranberry juice on urinary and nonurinary bacterial isolates. *Microbios* 55: 173–181, 224–225, 1988.

3. Zafriri D, et al. Inhibitory activity of cranberry juice on adherence of type 1 and type P fimbriated *Escherichia coli* to eucaryotic cells. *Antimicrob Agents Chemother* 33(1): 92–98, 1989.

4. Avorn J, et al. Reduction of bacteriuria and pyuria after ingestion of cranberry juice. *JAMA* 271: 751–754, 1994.

5. Schaefer AJ. Recurrent urinary tract infections in the female patient. *Urology* 32(Suppl.): 12–15, 1988.

Damiana

1. Willard T. The wild rose scientific herbal. Calgary, Canada: Wild Rose College of Natural Healing, Ltd., 1991: 104–105.

2. Duke JA. CRC handbook of medicinal herbs. Boca Raton, FL: CRC Press, 1985: 492.

3. Newall C, et al. Herbal medicines: A guide for health-care professionals. London: Pharmaceutical Press, 1996: 94.

Dandelion

1. Susnik F. Present state of knowledge of the medicinal plant *Taraxacum officinale* Weber. *Med Razgledi* 21: 323–328, 1982.

2. Racz-Kotilla, et al. The action of *Taraxacum officinale* extracts on the body weight and diureses of laboratory animals. *Planta Med* 26: 212–217, 1974.

3. Newall C, et al. Herbal medicines: A guide for health-care professionals. London: Pharmaceutical Press, 1996: 96.

Devil's Claw

1. Lecomte A, et al. *Harpagophytum* dans l'arthrose: Etude en double insu contre placebo. *Le Magazine* 15: 27–30, 1992.

2. ESCOP monograph. Fascicule 2: *Harpagophyti radix*. Exeter, UK: ESCOP, 1997.

3. Chrubasik S, et al. Effectiveness of *Harpagophytum procumbens* in treatment of acute low back pain. *Phytomedicine* 3(1): 1–10, 1996.

4. Schulz V, et al. Rational phytotherapy. New York: Springer-Verlag, 1998: 263.

5. ESCOP. 1997.

6. Moussard C, et al. A drug used in traditional medicine, *Harpagophytum procumbens*: No evidence for NSAID-like effect on whole blood eicosonoid production in humans. *Prostaglandins Leukot Essent Fatty Acids* 46: 283–286, 1992.

7. ESCOP. 1997.

Dong Quai

1. Chang HM, et al. Pharmacology and application of Chinese materia medica. Singapore: World Scientific, 1983.

2. Igarashi M. Proceedings of the satellite symposium on Sino-Japanese traditional medicine (Kampo). 16th World International Congress on Pharmacology. Excerpta Medica, 1987: 141–143.

3. Bensky D and Gamble A. Chinese herbal medicine: Materia medica. Seattle, WA: Eastland Press, 1986.

4. Hsu HY, et al. Oriental materia medica: A concise guide. Long Beach, CA: Oriental Healing Arts Institute, 1986: 540–542.

5. Zhu D. Dong quai. *Am J Chin Med* 90(3–4): 117–125, 1987.

6. Hirata JD, et al. Does dong quai have estrogenic effects in postmenopausal women? A double-blind placebo-controlled trial. *Fertil Steril* 68(6): 981–986, 1997.

7. Chang HM, et al. 1983.

8. Igarashi M. 1987.

9. Bensky D and Baronet R. Chinese herbal medicine formulas and strategies. Seattle, WA: Eastland Press, 1990.

10. Chang HM, et al. 1983.

11. Bensky D and Baronet R. 1990.

12. Zhu D. Dong quai. 1987.

Echinacea

1. Dorn M. Milderung grippaler Effekte durch ein pflanzliches Immunstimulans. Natur- und Ganzheitsmedizin. As cited in Schulz V, et al. Rational phytotherapy. New York: Springer-Verlag, 1998: 277.

2. Braunig B, et al. *Echinacea purpurea* root for strengthening the immune response in flu-like infections. *Z Phytother* 13: 7–13, 1992.

3. Dorn M, et al. Placebo-controlled double-blind study of *Echinacea pallidae radix* in upper respiratory tract infections. *Complement Ther Med* 3: 40–42, 1997.

4. Hoheisel O, et al. Echinagard treatment shortens the course of the common cold: A double-blind placebo-controlled clinical trial. *Eur J of Clin Res* 9: 261–268, 1997.

5. Melchart MD, et al. Echinacea root extracts for the prevention of upper respiratory tract infections. A double-blind placebo-controlled randomized trial. *Arch Fam Med* 7: 541–545, 1998.

6. Melchart D, et al. Immunomodulation with echinacea—A systematic review of controlled clinical trials. *Phytomedicine* 1: 245–254, 1994.

7. Bauer R, et al. Echinacea species as potential immunostimulatory drugs. *Econ Med Plant Res* 5: 253–321, 1991.

8. Wagner V, et al. Immunostimulating polysaccharides (heteroglycans) of higher plants. *Arzneimittelforschung* 35: 1069–1075, 1985.

9. Stimpel M, et al. Macrophage activation and induction of macrophage cytotoxicity by purified polysaccharide fractions from the plant *Echinacea purpurea. Infect Immun* 46: 845–849, 1984.

10. Luettig B, et al. Macrophage activation by the polysaccharide arabinogalactan isolated from plant cell cultures of *Echinacea purpurea. J Natl Cancer Inst* 81: 669–675, 1989.

11. Mose J. Effect of echinacin on phagocytosis and natural killer cells. *Med Welt* 34: 1463–1467, 1983.

12. Vomel V. Influence of a non-specific immune stimulant on phagocytosis of erythrocytes and ink by the reticuloendothelial system of isolated perfused rat livers of different ages. *Arzneimittelforschung* 34: 691–695, 1984.

13. Hobbs C. The echinacea handbook. Portland, OR: Eclectic Medical Publications, 1989.

14. Schulz V, et al. Rational phytotherapy. New York: Springer-Verlag, 1998: 278.

15. Bergner P. Goldenseal and the common cold: The antibiotic myth. *Med Herbalism* 8(4): 1–10, 1997.

16. Schulz V, et al. 1998: 276.

17. Mengs U, et al. Toxicity of *Echinacea purpurea* acute, subacute, and genotoxicity studies. *Arzneimittelforschung Drug Res* 41(11): 1076–1081, 1991.

18. Parnham MJ. Benefit-risk assessment of the squeezed sap of the purple coneflower *(echinacea purpurea)* for long-term oral immunostimulation. *Phytomedicine* 3(1): 99–102, 1996.

19. Parnham MJ. 1996.

Elderberry

1. Zakay-Rones Z, et al. Inhibition of several strains of influenza virus and reduction of symptoms by an elderberry

extract (*Sambucus nigra* L.) during an outbreak of influenza B Panama. *J Altern Complement Med* 1(4): 361–369, 1995.

2. Shapira-Nahor B, et al. The effect of Sambucol® on HIV infection in vitro. Annual Israel Congress of Microbiology, February 6–7, 1995.

3. Morag A, et al. Inhibition of sensitive and acyclovir-resistant HSV-1 strains by an elderberry extract in vitro. Xth International Congress of Virology, Abstract 18–23 (Jerusalem, 1996).

Elecampane

1. Reiter M, et al. Relaxant effects on tracheal and ileal smooth muscles of the guinea pig. *Arzneimittelforschung* 35: 408–414, 1985.

2. Newall C, et al. Herbal medicines: A guide for health-care professionals. London: Pharmaceutical Press, 1996: 106.

Ephedra

1. Blumenthal M. A review of the botany, chemistry, medicinal uses, safety concerns, and legal status of ephedra and its alkaloids. *Herbal Gram* 34: 22–57, 1995.

2. Physicians' desk reference for herbal medicines. Montvale, NJ: Medical Economics Company, Inc., 1998: 827.

Evening Primrose

1. Horrobin DF. Nutritional and medical importance of gamma-linolenic acid. *Prog Lipid Res* 31: 163–194, 1992.

2. Pye JK, et al. Clinical experience of drug treatment for mastalgia. *Lancet* ii: 373–377, 1985.

3. Horrobin DF, et al. Abnormalities in plasma essential fatty acid levels in women with premenstrual syndrome and with nonmalignant breast disease. *J Nutr Med* 2: 259–264, 1991.

4. Pashby N, et al. A clinical trial of EPO and mastalgia. *Br J Surg* 68: 801–824, 1981.

5. Budeiri D, et al. Is evening primrose oil of value in the treatment of premenstrual syndrome? *Controlled Clinical Trials* 17: 60–68, 1996.

6. Stevens EJ, et al. Essential fatty acid treatment prevents nerve ischaemia and associated conduction anomalies in rats

with experimental diabetes mellitus. *Diabetologia* 36(5): 397–401, 1993.

7. Reichert RG. Evening primrose oil and diabetic neuropathy. *Q Rev Natl Med* Summer: 141–145, 1995.

8. Keen H, et al. Treatment of diabetic neuropathy with gamma-linolenic acid. The gamma-linolenic acid multicenter trial group. *Diabetes Care* 16(1): 8–15, 1993.

9. Horrobin DF. The use of gamma-linolenic acid in diabetic neuropathy. *Agents Actions Suppl* 37: 120–144, 1992.

10. Hederos CA, et al. Epogam evening primrose oil treatment in atopic dermatitis and asthma. *Arch Dis Child* 75(6): 494–497, 1996.

11. Morse PF, et al. Meta-analysis of placebo-controlled studies of the efficacy of Epogam in the treatment of atopic eczema. Relationship between plasma essential fatty acid changes and clinical response. *Br J Dermatol* 121(1): 75–90, 1989.

12. Horrobin DF. 1992.

13. Horrobin DF, et al. Gamma-linolenic acid: An intermediate in essential fatty acid metabolism with potential as an ethical pharmaceutical and as a food. *Rev Contemp Pharmacother* 1: 1–45, 1990.

14. Horrobin DF. Essential fatty acids in the management of impaired nerve function in diabetes. *Diabetes* 46(Suppl. 2): S90–S93, 1997.

15. Vaddad KS. The use of gamma-linolenic acid and linoleic acid to differentiate between temporal lobe epilepsy and schizophrenia. *Prostaglandins Med* 6: 375–379, 1981.

16. Horrobin DF. The regulation of prostaglandin biosynthesis by the manipulation of essential fatty acid metabolism. *Rev Pure Appl Pharmacol* 4: 339–383, 1983.

Eyebright

1. Lawrence Review of Natural Products. Eyebright monograph. St. Louis, MO: Facts and Comparisons Division, J.B. Lipincott Company, 1996.

2. Duke JA. CRC handbook of medicinal herbs. Boca Raton, FL: CRC Press, 1985: 141.

Fenugreek

1. Sharma RD, et al. Use of fenugreek seed powder in the management of non-insulin dependent diabetes mellitus. *Nutr Res* 16:1331–1339, 1996.

2. Madar Z, et al. Glucose-lowering effect of fenugreek in non-insulin dependent diabetics. *Eur J Clin Nutr* 42: 51–54, 1988.

3. Sharma RD, Raghuram TC, and Rao NS. Effect of fenugreek seeds on blood glucose and serum lipids in type I diabetes. *Eur J Clin Nutr* 44: 301–306, 1990.

4. Leung A, et al. Encyclopedia of common natural ingredients used in food, drugs, and cosmetics. New York: John Wiley and Sons, 1996: 243–244.

Feverfew

1. Castleman, M. The healing herbs. Emmaus, PA: Rodale Press, 1991: 173–176.

2. Johnson ES, et al. Efficacy of feverfew as a prophylactic treatment of migraine. *Br Med J* 291: 569–573, 1985.

3. Bohlmann F, et al. Sesquiterpene lactones and other constituents from *Tanacetum parthenium*. *Phytochemistry* 21: 2543–2549, 1982.

4. Makheja AM, et al. The active principle in feverfew. *Lancet* ii: 1054, 1981.

5. Makheja AM, et al. A platelet phospholipase inhibitor from the medicinal herb feverfew (*Tanacetum parthenium*). *Prostaglandins Leukotr Med* 8: 653–660, 1982.

6. Heptinstall S, et al. Extracts from feverfew inhibit granule secretion in blood platelets and polymorphonuclear leukocytes. *Lancet* 8437: 1071–1074, 1985.

7. Tyler V. Herbs of choice. New York: Pharmaceutical Products Press, 1994: 127.

8. De Weerdt CJ, et al. Herbal medicines in migraine prevention. Randomized double-blind placebo controlled crossover trial of a feverfew preparation. *Phytomedicine* 3(3): 225–230, 1996.

9. Murphy JS, et al. Randomized, double-blind, placebo-controlled trial of feverfew in migraine prevention. *Lancet* 23: 189–192, 1988.

10. Palevitch DG, et al. Feverfew (*Tanacetum parthenium*) as a prophylactic treatment for migraine: A double-blind, placebo-controlled study. *Phytomed Res* 11(7): 506–511, 1997.

11. De Weerdt CJ, et al. 1996.

12. Newall C. Herbal medicines: A guide for health-care professionals. London: Pharmaceutical Press, 1996: 120.

13. Murphy JS, et al. 1988.

14. Johnson ES, et al. 1985.

15. Johnson ES, et al. 1985.

Garlic

1. Efendi JL, et al. The effect of the aged garlic extract, "Kyolic," on the development of experimental atherosclerosis. *Atherosclerosis* 132(1): 37–42, 1997.

2. Schulz V, et al. Rational phytotherapy. New York: Springer-Verlag, 1998: 112.

3. Quereshi AA, et al. Inhibition of cholesterol and fatty acid biosynthesis in liver enzymes and chicken hepatocytes by polar fractions of garlic. *Lipids* 18: 343–348, 1983.

4. Gebhardt R. Multiple inhibitory effects of garlic extracts on cholesterol biosynthesis in hepatocytes. *Lipids* 28(6): 613–619, 1993.

5. Gebhardt R, et al. Inhibition of cholesterol biosynthesis by allicin and ajoene in rat hepatocytes and HepG2 cells. *Biochem Biophys Acta* 1213: 57–62, 1994.

6. Schulz V, et al. 1998: 113.

7. Agarwal KC, et al. Therapeutic actions of garlic constituents. *Med Res Rev* 16(1): 111–124, 1996.

8. Legnani C, et al. Effects of dried garlic preparation on fibrinolysis and platelet aggregation in health subjects. *Arzneimittelforschung* 43: 119–121, 1993.

9. Chutani SK, et al. The effect of dried vs. raw garlic on fibrinolytic activity in man. *Atherosclerosis* 38: 417–421, 1981.

10. Kiesewetter H, et al. Effect of garlic on thrombocyte aggregation, microcirculation, and other risk factors. *Int J Clin Pharmacol Ther Toxicol* 29: 151–155, 1991.

11. Reuter HD, et al. *Allium sativum* and *Allium ursinum:* Chemistry, pharmacology, and medical applications. *Econ Med Plant Res* 6: 56–108, 1994.

12. Popov I, et al. Antioxidant effects of aqueous garlic extract, 1st communication: Direct detection using photochemoluminescence. *Arzneimittelforschung Drug Res* 44(1): 602–604, 1994.

13. Torok B, et al. Effectiveness of garlic on radical activity in radical generating systems. *Arzneimittelforschung Drug Res* 44(1): 608–611, 1994.

14. Silagy CA, et al. A meta-analysis of the effect of garlic on blood pressure. *J Hypertens* 12(4): 463–468, 1994.

15. Warshafsky S, et al. Effect of garlic on total serum cholesterol. A meta-analysis. *Ann Intern Med* 119(7) Part 1: 599–605.

16. Mader FH. Treatment of hyperlipidaemia with garlic-powder tablets. Evidence from the German Association of General Practitioners' multicentric placebo-controlled double-blind study. *Arzneimittelforschung* 40(10): 1111–1116, 1990.

17. Steiner M, et al. A double-blind crossover study in moderately hypercholesterolemic men that compared the effect of aged garlic extract and placebo administration on blood lipids. *Am J Clin Nutr* 64(6): 866–870, 1996.

18. Holzgartner H, et al. Comparison of the efficacy and tolerance of a garlic preparation vs. bezafibrate. *Arzneim Forsch* 42(12): 1473–1477, 1992.

19. Neil HA, et al. Garlic powder in the treatment of moderate hyperlipidaemia: A controlled trial and meta-analysis. *J R Coll Physicians Lond* 30(4): 329–334, 1996.

20. Simons LA, et al. On the effect of garlic on plasma lipids and lipoproteins in mild hypercholesterolaemia. *Atherosclerosis* 113(2): 219–225, 1995.

21. Santos OS de A, et al. Effects of garlic powder and garlic oil preparations on blood lipids, blood pressure and well being. *Br J Clin Res* 6: 91–100, 1995.

22. Silagy CA, et al. 1994.

23. Schulz V, et al. Rational phytotherapy. New York: Springer-Verlag, 1998: 119.

24. Auer W, et al. Hypertension and hyperlipidemia: Garlic helps in mild cases. *Br J Clin Pract Symp* 69 (Suppl.): 3–6, 1990.

25. Santos, OS de A., et al. 1995.

26. Breithaupt-Grogler K, et al. Protective effect of chronic garlic intake on the elastic properties of the aorta in the elderly. *Circulation* 96(7): 2649–2655, 1997.

27. Bordia A. Knoblauch und koronare Herzkrankheit: Wirkungen einer Dreijahrigen Behandlung mit Knoblauchextrakt auf die Reinfarkt-und Mortalitatsrate. *Dtsch Apoth Ztg* 129(Suppl. 15): 16–17. As reported in the ESCOP monographs. Fascicule 3: *Allii sativi bulbus* (garlic). Exeter, UK: ESCOP, 1997: 4.

28. Steinmetz KA, et al. Vegetables, fruit and colon cancer in the Iowa Women's Health Study. *Am J Epidemiol* 139(1): 1–13, 1994.

29. Ernst E. Can allium vegetables prevent cancer? *Phytomedicine* 4(1): 79–83, 1997.

30. Agarwal KC, et al. 1996.

31. Nagai K. Experimental studies on the preventive effect of garlic extract against infection with influenza virus. *Jpn J Infect Dis* 47: 321, 1973.

32. Chowdhury AK, et al. Efficacy of aqueaous extract of garlic and allicin in experimental shigellosis in rabbits. *Indian J Med Res* 93: 33–36, 1991.

33. Sharma VD, et al. Antibacterial property of *Alltum sativum* Linn.: In vivo and in vitro studies. *Indian J Exp Biol* 15(6): 466–468, 1977.

34. Hunan Hospital. Garlic in cryptococcal meningitis. A preliminary report of 21 cases. *Chin Med J* 93: 123–126, 1980.

35. Caporaso N, et al. Antifungal activity in human urine and serum after ingestion of garlic (*Allium sativum*). *Antimicrob Agents Chemother* 23(5): 700–702, 1983.

36. Sumiyoshi H, et al. Chronic toxicity test of garlic extracts in rats. *J Toxicol Sci* 9: 61–75, 1984.

37. Schulz V, et al. 1998: 121.

38. Schulz V, et al. 1998: 121.

Gentian

1. Lininger S, et al. The natural pharmacy. Rocklin, CA: Prima Publishing, 1998: 267.

2. Newall C, et al. Herbal medicines: A guide for health-care professionals. London: Pharmaceutical Press, 1996: 134.

Ginger

1. Tyler V. Herbs of choice. New York: Haworth Press, 1994: 42.

2. Holtman S, et al. The anti-motion sickness mechanism of ginger. *Acta Otolaryngol* 108: 168–174, 1989.

3. Mowrey DB. Motion sickness, ginger, and psychophysics. *Lancet* i: 655–657, 1982.

4. ESCOP monographs. Fascicule 1: *Zingiberis rhizoma.* Exeter, UK: ESCOP, 1997.

5. Grontved A, et al. Ginger root against seasickness. A controlled trial on the open sea. *Acta Otolaryngol (Stockh)* 105: 45–49, 1988.

6. Stott JRR, et al. A double-blind comparative trial of powdered ginger root, hyosine (sic) hydrobromide and cinnarizine in the prophylaxis of motion sickness induced by cross coupled stimulation. Advisory Group for Aerospace Research and Development, Conference Proceedings 372 (39):1–6, 1985.

7. Stewart JJ, et al. Effects of ginger on motion sickness susceptibility and gastric function. *Pharmacology* 42: 111–120, 1991.

8. Wood CD, et al. Comparison of efficacy of ginger with various antimotion sickness drugs. *Clin Res Pract Drug Reg Aff* 6:129–136, 1988.

9. Fischer-Rasmussen W, et al. Ginger treatment of hyperemesis gravidarum. *Eur J Obstet Gynecol Reprod Biol* 38: 19–24, 1990.

10. Bone ME, et al. Ginger root: A new anti-emetic. The effect of ginger root on postoperative nausea and vomiting after major gynecological surgery. *Anaesthesia* 45: 669–671, 1990.

11. Phillips S, et al. *Zingiber officinale* (ginger)—An anti-emetic for day case surgery. *Anaesthesia* 48: 715–717, 1993.

12. Arfeen Z, et al. A double-blind randomized controlled trial of ginger for the prevention of postoperative nausea and vomiting. *Anaesth Intensive Care* 23(4): 449–452, 1995.

13. Visalyaputra S, et al. The efficacy of ginger root in the prevention of postoperative nausea and vomiting after outpatient gynaecological laparoscopy. *Anaesthesia* 53: 506–510 1998.

14. Srivastava KC. Isolation and effects of some ginger components on platelet aggregation and eicosanoid biosynthesis. *Prostaglandins Leukot Med* 25: 187–198, 1986.

15. Srivastava K. Effects of aqueous extracts of onion, garlic, and ginger on the platelet aggregation and metabolism of arachidonic acid in the blood vascular system: In vitro study. *Prostaglandins Leukot Med* 13: 227–235, 1984.

16. Srivastava KC. Effect of onion and ginger consumption on platelet thromboxane production in humans. *Prostaglandins Leukot Essent Fatty Acids* 35: 183–185, 1989.

17. Janssen PL, et al. Consumption of ginger (*Zingiber officinale Roscoe*) does not affect ex vivo platelet thromboxane production in humans. *Eur J Clin Nutr* 50(11): 772–774, 1996.

18. Bordia A, et al. Effect of ginger (*Zingiber officinale Rosc.*) and fenugreek (*Trigonella foenumgraecum* L.) on blood lipids, blood sugar and platelet aggregation in patients with coronary artery disease. *Prostaglandins Leukot Essent Fatty Acids* 56(5): 379–384, 1997.

19. Lumb AB. Effect of dried ginger on human platelet function. *Thromb Haemost* 71: 110–111, 1994.

Ginkgo

1. Schulz V, et al. Rational phytotherapy. New York: Springer-Verlag, 1998: 288–292.

2. Tamborini A, et al. Value of standardized *Ginkgo biloba* extract (EGb761) in the management of congestive symptoms

of premenstrual syndrome. *Rev Fr Gynecol Obstet* 88: 447–457, 1993.

3. Schulz V, et al. 1998: 41.

4. Jung F, et al. Effect of *Ginkgo biloba* on fluidity of blood and peripheral microcirculation in volunteers. *Arzneimittelforschung Drug Res* 40: 589–593, 1990.

5. De Feudis FV. *Ginkgo biloba* extract (EGb 761): Pharmacological activities and clinical applications. Paris: Elsevier, 1991: 143–146.

6. Kleijnen J and Knipschild P. *Ginkgo biloba. Lancet* 340: 1136–1139, 1992.

7. Schulz V, et al. 1998: 41.

8. Kleijnen J and Knipschild P. 1992.

9. Kanowski S, et al. Proof of efficacy of the *Ginkgo biloba* special extract EGb 761 in outpatients suffering from mild to moderate primary degenerative dementia of the Alzheimer type or multi-infarct dementia. *Pharmacopsychiatry* 29: 47–56, 1996.

10. Hofferberth B. The efficacy of EGb 761 in patients with senile dementia of the Alzheimer type, a double-blind, placebo-controlled study on different levels of investigation. *Hum Psychopharmacol* 9: 215–222, 1994.

11. Schulz V, et al. 1998: 46.

12. LeBars PL, et al. A placebo-controlled, double-blind, randomized trial of an extract of *Ginkgo biloba* for dementia. *JAMA* 278: 1327–1332, 1997.

13. Schulz V, et al. 1998: 126.

14. Peters H, Kieser M, and Holscher U. Demonstration of the efficacy of *Ginkgo biloba* special extract EGb 761 on intermittent claudication—A placebo-controlled double-blind multicenter trial. *Vasa* 27: 106–110, 1998.

15. Blume J, Kieser M, and Holscher U. Placebo-controlled double-blind study of the effectiveness of *Ginkgo biloba* special extract EGb 761 in trained patients with intermittent claudication (Engl Abst Only). *Vasa* 25: 265–274, 1996.

16. Tamborini A, et al. 1993.

17. Lebuisson DA, et al. Treatment of senile macular degeneration with *Ginkgo biloba* extract: A preliminary double-blind, drug vs. placebo study. *Presse Med* 15: 1556–1558, 1986.

18. Cohen A, et al. Treatment of sexual dysfunction with *Ginkgo biloba* extract. Scientific Reports—Paper session from the proceedings of the APA annual meeting. 1997.

19. De Feudis FV. 1991.

20. De Feudis FV. 1991.

21. Schulz V, et al. 1998: 247.

22. Rosenblatt M and Mindel J. Spontaneous hyphema associated with ingestion of *Ginkgo biloba* extract. *N Engl J Med* 336(15): 1108, 1997.

23. Rowin J and Lewis SL. Spontaneous bilateral subdural hematomas associated with chronic *Ginkgo biloba* ingestion. *Neurology* 46: 1775–1776, 1996.

Ginseng

1. Schulz V, et al. Rational phytotherapy. New York: Springer-Verlag, 1998: 271, 273.

2. Brekhman II. *Eleutheroccoccus:* 20 years of research and clinical application. Presented at the 1st International symposium on *eleutherococcus*, Hamburg, Germany, 1980. In Brown D. Herbal prescriptions for better health. Rocklin, CA: Prima Publishing, 1997.

3. Brekhman II. *Eleutherococcus:* Clinical data. USSR Foreign Trade Publication. Medexport, 1970. In Brown D. Herbal prescriptions for better health. Rocklin, CA: Prima Publishing 1997.

4. Sonnenborn U, et al. Ginseng (*Panax ginseng* C.A. Meyer). *Z Phytother* 11: 35–49, 1990.

5. Schulz V, et al. 1998.

6. Scaglione F, et al. Efficacy and safety of the standardised ginseng extract G115 for potentiating vaccination against the influenza syndrome and protection against the common cold. *Drugs Exp Clin Res* 22(2): 65–72, 1996.

7. Sotaneimi EA, et al. Ginseng therapy in non-insulin–dependent diabetic patients. *Diabetes Care* 18(10): 1373–1375, 1995.

8. Sorenson H, et al. A double-masked study of the effects of ginseng on cognitive functions. *Curr Ther Res Clin Exp* 57(12): 959–968, 1996.

9. Dowling EA, et al. Effect of *Eleutherococcus senticosus* on submaximal and maximal exercise performance. *Med Sci Sports Exerc* 28(4): 482–489, 1996.

10. Awang, DVC. Maternal use of ginseng and neonatal andiogenization. *JAMA* 266: 363, 1991.

11. Ploss E. *Panax ginseng.* C. A. Meyer. Scientific report. Cologne: Kooperation Phytopharmaka, 1988.

12. Lawrence Review of Natural Products. Ginseng monograph. St. Louis, Missouri. Facts and Comparisons Division, J.B. Lipincott Company, 1990.

13. Tyler V. Herbs of choice. New York: Haworth Press, 1994.

14. Siegel RK. *JAMA* 241: 1614–1615, 1979.

15. Tyler V. 1994.

16. Schulz V, et al. 1998.

Goldenrod

1. Tyler V. Herbs of choice. New York: Haworth Press, 1994: 74–75.

2. ESCOP monographs. Fascicule 2: *Solidaginis virgaureae herba.* Exeter, UK: ESCOP, 1996: 1–3.

3. ESCOP monographs. 1996: 2

4. ESCOP monographs. 1996: 2

Goldenseal

1. Hahn FE, et al. Berberine. *Antibiotics* 3: 577–588, 1976.

2. Amin AH, et al. Berberine sulfate: Antimicrobial activity, bioassay, and mode of action. *Can J Microbiol* 15: 1067–1076, 1969.

3. Bensky D and Gamble H. Chinese herbal medicine: Materia medica. Seattle, WA: Eastland Press, 1986.

4. Bergner P. The healing power of echinacea and goldenseal. Rocklin, CA: Prima Publishing, 1997.

5. Bergner P. 1997.

6. Foster S. Botanical Series No. 309—Goldenseal. Austin, TX: American Botanical Council, 1991: 5–6.

7. DeSmet PAGM, et al., eds. Adverse effects of herbal drugs. Berlin: Springer-Verlag, 1992: 97–104.

Gotu Kola

1. Kartnig T. Clinical applications of *Centella asiatica* (L.) Urb. *Herbs Spices Med Plants* 3: 146–173, 1988.

2. Nalini K, et al. Effect of *Centella asiatica* fresh leaf aqueous extract on learning and memory and biogenic amine turnover in albino rats. *Fitoterapia* 63(3): 232–237, 1992.

3. Cesarone MR, et al. Activity of *Centella asiatica* in venous insufficiency. *Minerva Cardioangiol* 42: 137–143, 1992.

4. Cesarone MR, et al. The microcirculatory activity of *Centella asiatica* in venous insufficiency. A double-blind study. *Minerva Cardioangiol* 42: 299–304, 1994.

5. Murray M. The healing power of herbs. Rocklin, CA: Prima Publishing, 1995: 177.

6. Kartnig T. 1988.

7. Laerum OD, et al. Reticuloses and epidermal tumors in hairless mice after topical skin applications of cantharidin and asiaticoside. *Cancer Res* 32: 1463–1469, 1972.

8. Bosse JP, et al. Clinical study of a new antikeloid drug. *Ann Plast Surg* 3: 13–21, 1979.

9. Basellini A, et al. Varicose disease in pregnancy. *Ann Obstet Gyn Med Perinat* 106: 337–341, 1985.

Grape Seed PCOs

1. Schwitters B, et al. OPC in practice. Bioflavanols and their applications. Rome, Italy: Alfa Omega, 1993.

2. Masquelier J, et al. Stabilization of collagen by procyanidolic oligomers. *Acta Ther* 7: 101–105, 1981.

3. Masquelier J. Procyanidolic oligomers. *J Parums Cosm Arom* 95: 89–97, 1990.

4. Tixier JM, et al. Evidence by in vivo and in vitro studies that binding of pycnogenols to elastin affects its rate of degradation by elastases. *Biochem Pharmacol* 33: 3933–3939, 1984.

5. Facino RM, et al. Free radical scavenging action and anti-enzyme activities of procyanidines from *Vitis vinifera*. A mechanism for their capillary protective action. *Arzneimittelforschung* 44: 592–601, 1994.

6. Kuttan R, et al. Collagen treated with catechin becomes resistant to the action of mammalian collagenase. *Experientia* 37: 221–223, 1981.

7. Masquelier J, et al. 1981.

8. Bombardelli E, et al. *Vitis vinifera* L. *Fitoterapia* 66: 291–317, 1995.

9. Henriet, JP. Exemplary study for a phleboteropic substance, the EIVE study. On file with Primary Services International, Southport, CT.

10. Delacroix P, et al. Double-blind study of endotelon in chronic venous insufficiency. *La Revue de Medecine* (Eng Abst Only) 27–28, 31: 1793–1802.

11. Pecking A, et al. Oligomeric proanthocyanidins (endotelons) in the treatment of post-therapeutic lympedema in the upper limbs (Eng Abst Only). Association de Lymphologie de Lange Française, Hôpital Saint-Louis, 75010, Paris, France 69–73, 1989.

12. Baruch J. Effect of endotelon in post-surgical edemas (Eng Abst Only). *Ann Chir Plast Esthet* 29 (4): 393–395, 1984.

13. Parienti JJ, et al. Post-traumatic edemas in sports: A controlled test of endotelon (Eng Abst Only). *Gaz Med France* 90 (3): 231–236.

14. Corbe C, et al. Light vision and chorioretinal circulation. Study of the effect of procyanidolic oligomers (endotelon). *J Fr Ophtalmol* 11: 453–460, 1988.

15. Boissin JP, et al. Chorioretinal circulation and dazzling: Use of procyanidol oligomers. *Bull Soc Ophtamol Fr* 88: 173–174, 177–179, 1988.

16. Schwitters B, et al. 1993.

17. Wegrowski J, et al. The effect of procyanidolic oligomers on the composition of normal and hypercholesterolemic rabbit aortas. *Biochem Pharmacol* 33: 3491–3497, 1984.

18. Uchida S, et al. Condensed tannins scavenge active free radicals. *Med Sci Res* 15: 831–832, 1987.

19. Cendre P. Effet protecteur des oligomeres procyandiloques sur le lathyrisme experimental chez le rat. *Ann Pharm Fr* 43(1): 61–71, 1985.

20. Schulz V, et al. Rational phytotherapy. New York: Springer-Verlag, 1998: 282–284.

Green Tea

1. Snow J. Herbal monograph: *Camellia sinensi* (L.) Kuntze (Theaceae) protocol. *J Botanical Medicine* Autumn: 47–51, 1995.

2. Imai K, et al. Cancer-preventive effects of drinking green tea among a Japanese population. *Prev Med* 26(6): 769–775, 1997.

3. Kohlmeier L, et al. Tea and cancer prevention: An evaluation of the epidemiologic literature. *Nutr Cancer* 27(1): 1–13, 1997.

Guggul

1. Satyavati GV. Gum guggul (*Commiphor mukul*)—The success story of an ancient insight leading to a modern discovery. *Indian J Med Res* 87: 327–335, 1988.

2. Nityanand S, et al. Clinical trials with gugulipid. A new hypolipidaemic agent. *J Assoc Physicians India* 37(5): 323–328, 1989.

3. Agarwal RC, et al. Clinical trial of gugulipid a new hyperlipidemic agent of plant origin in primary hyperlipidemia. *Indian J Med Res* 84: 626–634, 1986.

4. Nityanand S, et al. 1989.

5. Agarwal RC, et al. 1986.

6. Satyavati GV. 1988.

7. Newall C, et al. Herbal medicines: A guide for health-care professionals. London: Pharmaceutical Press, 1996: 200.

Gymnema

1. Lininger S, et al. The natural pharmacy. Rocklin, CA: Prima Publishing, 1998: 276

2. Lawrence Review of Natural Products. Gymnema monograph. St. Louis, MO: Facts and Comparisons Division, J.B. Lipincott Company, 1993.

3. Shanmugasundaram ERB, et al. Use of *Gymnema sylvestre* leaf extract in the control of blood glucose in insulin-dependent diabetes mellitus. *J Ethnopharmacol* 30: 281–294, 1990.

4. Baskaran K, et al. Antidiabetic effect of a leaf extract from *Gymnema sylvestre* in non-insulin–dependent diabetes mellitus patients. *J Ethnopharmacol* 30: 295–305, 1990.

Hawthorn

1. Popping S, et al. Effect of a hawthorn extract on contraction and energy turnover of isolated rat cardiomyocytes. *Arzneimittelforschung Drug Res* 45: 1157–1161, 1995.

2. Joseph G. Pharmacologic action profile of crataegus extract in comparison to epinephrine, amirinone, milrinone and digoxin in the isolated perfused guinea pig heart. *Arzneimittelforschung* 45(12): 1261–1265, 1995.

3. Schulz V, et al. Rational phytotherapy. New York: Springer-Verlag, 1998: 91–94.

4. Schulz V, et al. 1998: 91–95.

5. Ammon HTP, et al. Crataegus, toxicology, and pharmacology. *Planta Med* 43: 105–120, 209–239, 313–322, 1981.

6. Schulz V, et al. 1998: 97.

7. Tauchert M, et al. Crataegi folium cum flore bei herzinsuffizienz. As cited in Loew D, Tietbrock N, eds. Phytopharmaka in Forschung und klinischer Anwendung. Darmstadt: Steinkopff Verlag, 1995: 37–44.

8. Schulz V, et al. 1998: 90–98.

9. Tauchert M, et al. Weissdorn Extrakt als pflanzliches Cardiacum (Vorwort). Neubewertung der therapeutischen Wirksamkeit. *Munch Med Wschr* 136(Suppl. 1): 3–5, 1994.

10. Schulz V, et al. 1998: 95.

He Shou Wu

1. Chang HM. Pharmacology and applications of Chinese materia medica. World Scientific I: 620–624, 1986.

Hops

1. Schulz V, et al. Rational phytotherapy. New York: Springer-Verlag, 1998: 82–83.

2. Schulz V, et al. 1998: 83.

3. Duncan KL, et al. Malignant hyperthermia-like reaction secondary to ingestion of hops in five dogs. *J Am Vet Med Assoc* 210: 51–54, 1997.

Horse Chestnut

1. Newall C, et al. Herbal medicines: A guide for health-care professionals. London: Pharmaceutical Press, 1996: 166.

2. Kreysel HW, et al. A possible role of lysosomal enzymes in the pathogenesis of varicosis and the reduction in their serum activity by Venostatin. *Vasa* 12: 377–382, 1983.

3. Schulz V, et al. Rational phytotherapy. New York: Springer-Verlag, 1998: 131–134.

4. Neiss A, et al. Zum Wirksamkeitsnachweis von Rosskastaniensamenextrakt beim varikosen Symptomenkomplex. *Munch Med Wschr* 7: 213–216.

5. Diehm C, et al. Comparison of leg compression stocking and oral horse-chestnut seed extract therapy in patients with chronic venous insufficiency. *Lancet* 347: 292–294, 1996.

6. Schulz V, et al. 1998: 131.

7. Schulz V, et al. 1998: 131.

8. Newall C, et al. 1996: 166–167.

9. Schulz V, et al. 1998: 132.

Horsetail

1. Duke JA. CRC handbook of medicinal herbs. Boca Raton, FL: CRC Press, 1985: 492.

2. Fessenden RJ, et al. The biological properties of silicon compounds. *Adv Drug Res* 4: 95, 1987.

3. Weiss, R. Herbal medicine abstract arcanum. Gothenburg Sweden, 238–239, 1988.

4. Fabre B, et al. Thiaminase activity in *Equisetum arvense* and its extracts. *Planta Med Phytother* 26: 190–197, 1993.

5. Leung A, Foster S. Encyclopedia of common natural ingredients used in food, drugs, and cosmetics. New York: John Wiley and Sons, 1996: 307.

Juniper

1. Newall C, et al. Herbal medicines: A guide for health-care professionals. London: Pharmaceutical Press, 1996: 176.

2. Mascolo N, et al. Biological screening of Italian medicinal plants for anti-inflammatory activity. *Phytother Res* 1: 28–31, 1987.

3. Markkanen T, et al. Antiherpetic agent from juniper tree (*Juniperus cummunis*), its purification, identification, and testing in primary human amnion cell cultures. *Drugs Exp Clin Res* 7: 691–697, 1981.

4. Agarwal OP, et al. Antifertility effects of fruits of *Juniperus communis*. *Planta Med* 40(Suppl.): 98–101, 1980.

5. Newall C, et al. 1990: 176.

Kava

1. Meyer HJ, et al. Kawa-Pyrone-eine neuartige Substanz-gruppe zentraler Muskelrelaxantien vom Typ des Mephen-esins. *Klin Wschr* 44: 902–903, 1966.

2. Klohs MW, et al. A chemical and pharmacological investiga-tion of *Piper methysticum Forst*. *J Med Pharm Chem* 1: 95–103, 1959.

3. Bruggenmann F, et al. Die analgetische Wirkung der Kawa-Inhaltsstoffe Dihydrokawain und Dihydromethysticin. *Arzneimittelforschung* 13: 407–409, 1963.

4. Meyer HJ. Pharmakologie der Wirksamen Prinzipien des Kawa-Rhizoms (Piper methysticum Forst). *Arch Intern Pharmacodyn* 138: 505–535, 1962.

5. Meyer HJ. Lokalanaesthetische Eigenschaften naturlicher Kawa-Pyrone. *Arzneimittelforschung* 42: 407, 1964.

6. Meyer HJ, et al. 1966.

7. Singh YN. Effects of kava on neuromuscular transmission and muscle contractility. *J Ethnopharmacol* 7: 267–276, 1983.

8. Davies LP, et al. Kava pyrones and resin: Studies on GABA-A, GABA-B, and benzodiazepine binding sites in rodent brain. *Pharmacol Toxicol* 71(2): 120–126, 1992.

9. Jussofie A, Schmiz A, and Hiemke C. Kavapyrone enriched extract from *Piper methysticum* as modulator of the GABA binding site in different regions of rat brain. *Psychopharmacology* 116: 469–474, 1994.

10. Munte TF, et al. Effects of oxazepam and an extract of kava roots (*Piper methysticum*) on event-related potentials in a word recognition task. *Neuropsychobiology* 27(1): 46–53, 1993.

11. Heinze HJ, et al. Pharmacopsychological effects of oxazepam and kava extract in a visual search paradigm assessed with event-related potentials. *Pharmacopsychiatry* 27(6): 224–230, 1994.

12. Emser W and Bartylla K. Effect of kava extract WS 1490 on the sleep pattern in healthy subjects. *Neurol Psychiatr* 5: 636–642, 1991.

13. Volz HP, et al. Kava-kava extract WS 1490 versus placebo in anxiety disorders—A randomized placebo-controlled 25 week outpatient trial. *Pharmacopsychiatry* 30(1): 1–5, 1997.

14. Kinzler E, et al. Effect of a special kava extract in patients with anxiety, tension, and excitation states of non-psychotic genesis. Double-blind study with placebos over 4 weeks. *Arzneimittelforschung* 41(6): 584–588, 1991.

15. Warnecke G, et al. Wirksamkeit von Kawa-Kawa Extract beim klimakterischen Syndrom. *Z Phytother* 11: 81–86, 1990.

16. Warnecke G. Psychosomatic dysfunctions in the female climacteric. Clinical effectiveness and tolerance of kava extract WS 1490. *Fortschr Med* 109(4): 119–122, 1991.

17. Woelk H, et al. Behandlung von Angst-Patienten. *Z Allg Med* 69: 271–277, 1993.

18. Schulz V, et al. Rational phytotherapy. New York: Springer-Verlag, 1998: 68.

19. Schulz V, et al. 1998: 71.

20. Schulz V, et al. 1998: 71.

21. Norton SA, et al. Kava dermopathy. *Am Acad Dermatol* 31(1): 89–97, 1994.

22. Munte TF, et al. 1993.

23. Heinze HJ, et al. 1994.

24. Herberg KW. Effect of kava special extract WS 1490 combined with ethyl alcohol on safety-relevant performance parameters. *Blutalkohol* 30(2): 96–105, 1993.

25. Munte TF, et al. 1993.

26. Heinze HJ, et al. 1994.

27. Schulz V, et al. 1998: 72.

28. Duffield PH and Jamieson D. Development of tolerance to kava in mice. *Clin Experimental Pharmacology and Physiology* 18: 571–578, 1991.

29. Almeida JC and Grimsley EW. Coma from the health food store: Interaction between kava and alprazolam. *Ann Intern Med* 125(11): 940–941, 1996.

Kudzu

1. Keung WM, et al. Daidzin and daidzein suppress free choice ethanol intake by Syrian golden hamsters. *Proc Natl Acad Sci* 90: 10008–10012, 1993.

2. Overstreet DH. Suppression of alcohol intake after administration of the Chinese herbal medicine NPI-028 and its derivatives. *Alcohol Clin Exp Res* 20(2): 221–227, 1996.

Lapacho

1. Li CJ, et al. Beta-lapachone, a novel DNA topoisomerase I inhibitor with a mode of action different from camptothecin. *J Biol Chem* 268: 22463–22468, 1993.

2. Guiraud P, et al. Comparison of antibacterial and antifungal activities of lapachol and beta-lapachone. *Planta Med* 60: 373–374, 1994.

3. Oswald EH. Lapacho. *Br J Phytother* 4(3): 112–117, 1993.

Licorice

1. Newall C, et al. Herbal medicines: A guide for health-care professionals. London: Pharmaceutical Press, 1996: 183–184.

2. van Marle J, et al. Deglycyrrhizinised liquorice (DGL) and the renewal of rat stomach epithelium. *Eur J Pharmacol* 72: 219–25, 1981.

3. Johnson B and McIssac R. Effect of some anti-ulcer agents on mucosal blood flow. *Br J Pharmacol* 1: 308, 1981.

4. Schulz V, et al. Rational phytotherapy. New York: Springer-Verlag, 1998: 185.

5. Morgan AG, et al. Comparison between cimetidine and Caved-S in the treatment of gastric ulceration and subsequent maintenance therapy. *Gut* 23: 545–551, 1982.

6. Morgan AG, et al. Maintenance therapy: A two-year comparison between Caved-S and cimetidine treatment in the prevention of symptomatic gastric ulcer. *Gut* 26: 599–602, 1985.

7. Kassir ZA. Endoscopic controlled trial of four drug regimens in the treatment of chronic duodenal ulceration. *Ir Med J* 78: 153–156, 1985.

Maitake

1. Yamada Y, et al. Antitumor effect of orally administered extracts from fruit body of *Grifola frondosa* (maitake). *Chemotherapy* 38: 790–796, 1990.

2. Nanba H. Immunostimulant activity in vivo and anti-HIV activity in vitro of 3 branched b-1-6-glucans extracted from maitake mushrooms (*Grifola frondosa*). Amsterdam: VIII International Conference on AIDS, 1992 (Abstract).

Marshmallow

1. Newall C, et al. Herbal medicines: A guide for health-care professionals. London: Pharmaceutical Press, 1996: 188.

2. Tomodo M, et al. Hypoglycemic activity of twenty plant mucilages and three modified products. *Planta Med* 53: 8–12, 1987.

Melissa

1. Wolbling RH, et al. Clinical therapy of herpes simplex. *Therapiewoche* 34: 1193–1200, 1984.

2. Wolbling RH, et al. Local therapy of herpes simplex with dried extract from *Melisssa officinalis*. *Phytomedicine* 1: 25–31, 1994.

3. Dimitrova Z, et al. Antiherpes effect of *Melissa officinalis* L. extracts. *Acta Microbiol Bulg* 29: 65–72, 1993.

4. May S, et al. Antivirale Wirkung wassriger Pflanzenextrakte in Gewebekulturen. *Arzneimittelforschung Drug Res* 28: 1–7, 1978.

5. Wolbling RH, et al. 1994.

6. Wolbling RH, et al. 1984.

7. Wolbling RH, et al. 1994.

8. Wolbling RH, et al. 1984.

9. Wolbling RH, et al. 1994.

10. Wolbling RH, et al. 1994.

11. Isselbacher K, et al., eds. Harrison's principles of internal medicine, 13th ed. New York: McGraw Hill, 1994: 779.

12. Soulimani R, et al. Neurotropic action of the hydroalcoholic extract of *Melissa officinalis* in the mouse. *Planta Med* 57: 105–109, 1991.

13. Dressing H, et al. Insomnia: Are valerian/balm combinations of equal value to benzodiazepine? *Therapiewoche* 42: 726–736, 1992.

14. Wolbling RH, et al. 1994.

Milk Thistle

1. Schulz V, et al. Rational phytotherapy. New York: Springer-Verlag, 1998: 215.

2. Muriel P, et al. Silymarin protects against paracetamol-induced lipid peroxidation and liver damage. *J Appl Toxicol* 12: 6439–6442, 1992.

3. Paulova J, et al. Verification of the hepatoprotective and therapeutic effect of silymarin in experimental liver injury with tetrachloromethane in dogs. *Vet Med (Praha)* 35(10): 629–635, 1990.

4. Skakun NP, et al. Clinical pharmacology of Fegalon (review of the literature). *Vrach Delo* 5: 5–10, 1988.

5. Tuchweber B, et al. Prevention of silybin of phalloidin-induced acute hepatotoxicity. *Toxicol Appl Pharmacol* 51(2): 265–275, 1979.

6. Boari C, et al. Toxic occupational liver diseases. Therapeutic effects of silymarin. *Minerva Med* 72(40): 2679–2688, 1981.

7. Szilard S. Protective effect of Legalon in workers exposed to organic solvents. *Acta Med Hung* 45(2): 249–256, 1988.

8. Rui YC. Advances in pharmacological studies of silymarin. *Mem Inst Oswaldo Cruz* 86(Suppl. 2): 79–85, 1991.

9. Schulz V, et al. Rational phytotherapy. New York: Springer-Verlag, 1998: 216.

10. Hikino H, et al. Natural products for liver disease. As cited in Wagner H, et al. Economic and medicinal plant research, Vol 2. New York: Academic Press, 1988: 39–72.

11. Muzes G, et al. Effects of silymarin (Legalon) therapy on the antioxidant defense mechanism and lipid peroxidation in alcoholic liver disease (double-blind protocol). *Orv Hetil* 131(16): 863–866, 1990.

12. Giannola C, et al. A two-center study on the effects of silymarin in pregnant women and adult patients with so-called minor hepatic insufficiency. *Clin Ther* 114(2): 129–135, 1985.

13. Schulz V, et al. 1998: 218.

14. Berenguer J, et al. Double-blind trial of silymarin vs. placebo in the treatment of chronic hepatitis. *Munch Med Wochenschr* 119: 240–260, 1977.

15. Buzzelli G, et al. A pilot study on the liver protective effect of silybin-phosphatidylcholine complex (IdB 1016) in chronic active hepatitis. *Int J Clin Pharmacol Ther Toxicol* 31(9): 456–460, 1993.

16. Liruss F, et al. Cytoprotection in the nineties: Experience with ursodeoxycholic acid and silymarin in chronic liver disease. *Acta Physiol Hung* 80(1–4): 363–367, 1992.

17. Magliulo E, et al. Results of a double blind study on the effect of silymarin in the treatment of acute viral hepatitis, carried out at two medical centers. *Med Klin* 73: 28–29, 1060–1065, 1978.

18. Bode JC, et al. Silymarin for the treatment of acute viral hepatitis? Report of a controlled trial. *Med Klin* 72(12): 513–518, 1977.

19. Salmi H, et al. Effect of silymarin on chemical, functional and morphological alterations of the liver. *Scand J Gastroenterol* 17: 517–521, 1982.

20. Feher J. Liver protective action of silymarin therapy in chronic alcoholic liver diseases. *Orv Hetil* 130(51): 2723–2727, 1989.

21. Trinchet JC. Treatment of alcoholic hepatitis with silymarin. A double-blind comparative study in 116 patients. *Gastroenterol Clin Biol* 13(2): 120–124, 1989.

22. Bunout D, et al. Controlled study of the effect of silymarin on alcoholic liver disease. *Rev Med Chil* 120(12): 1370–1375, 1992.

23. Ferenci P, et al. Randomized controlled trial of silymarin treatment in patients with cirrhosis of the liver. *J Hepatol* 9: 105–113, 1989.

24. Pares A, et al. Effects of silymarin in alcoholic patients with cirrhosis of the liver: Results of a controlled, double-blind, randomized and multicenter trial. *J Hepatology* 28: 615–621, 1998.

25. Schandalik R, et al. Pharmacokinetics of silybin in bile following administration of silipide and silymarin in cholecsytectomy patients. *Arznneimittelforschung* 42(7): 964–968, 1992.

26. Barzaghi N, et al. Pharmacokinetic studies on IdB 1016, a silybin-phosphatidylcholine complex in health human subjects. *Eur J Drug Metab Pharmacokinet* 15(4): 333–338, 1990.

27. Awang D. Milk thistle. *Can Pharmacol J* 422: 403–404, 1993.

28. Albrecht M. Therapy of toxic liver pathologies with Legalon. *Z Klin Med* 47(2): 87–92, 1992.

29. Giannola C, et al. 1985.

Mullein

1. Tyler V. The honest herbal, 3rd ed. Binghamton, New York: Pharmaceutical Products Press, 1993: 219–220.

Neem

1. Charles V, et al. Village pharmacy. The neem tree yields products from pesticides to soap. *Sci Am* 44(1–2): 132, 1992.

2. Neem Foundation: www.neemfoundation.org

Nettle

1. Hryb DJ, et al. The effect of extracts of the roots of the stinging nettle (*Urtica dioica*) on the interaction of SHBG

with its receptor on human prostatic membranes. *Planta Med* 61: 31–32, 1995.

2. Wagner H, et al. Search for the antiprostatic principle of stinging nettle (*Urtica dioica*) roots. *Phytomedicine* 1: 213–224, 1994.

3. Schulz V, et al. Rational phytotherapy. New York: Springer-Verlag, 1998: 229.

4. ESCOP monographs. Fascicule 2: *Urticae radix*. Exter, UK: ESCOP, 2–4.

5. ESCOP. 1996: 4–5.

6. Dathe G, et al. Phytotherpie der beignen Prostatahyper-plasie (BPH). *Urologe B* 27: 223–226, 1987.

7. ESCOP. 1996: 4

8. ESCOP. 1996: 4

9. Mittman P. Randomized, double-blind study of freeze-dried *Urtica dioica* in the treatment of allergic rhinitis. *Planta Med* 56: 44–47, 1990.

10. ESCOP. 1996: 5.

Osha

1. Bensky D and Gamble A. Chinese herbal medicine: Materia medica. Seattle, WA: Eastland Press, 1986: 383–384.

2. Moore M. Medicinal plants of the mountain west. Santa Fe, NM: Museum of New Mexico Press, 1979: 119.

Passionflower

1. Schulz V, et al. Rational phytotherapy. New York: Springer-Verlag, 1998: 84.

2. Newall C, et al. Herbal medicines: A guide for health-care professionals. London: Pharmaceutical Press, 1996: 206.

Peppermint

1. Gunn JWC. The carminative action of volatile oils. *J Pharmacol Exp Ther* 16: 93–143, 1920.

2. Taylor BA, et al. Inhibitory effect of peppermint on gastrointestinal smooth muscle. *Gut* 24: 992, 1983.

3. Hawthorn M, et al. The actions of peppermint oil and menthol on calcium channel dependent processes in intestinal, neuronal and cardiac preparations. *Aliment Pharmcol Ther* 2: 101–118, 1988.

4. Rees WDW, et al. Treating irritable bowel syndrome with peppermint oil. *BMJ* ii: 835–836, 1979.

5. Dew MJ, et al. Peppermint oil for the irritable bowel syndrome: A multicentre trial. *Br J Clin Pract* 34: 55–57, 1989.

6. Nash P, et al. Peppermint oil does not relieve the pain of irritable bowel syndrome. *Br J Clin Pract* 40: 292–293, 1986.

7. Lawson MJ, et al. Failure of enteric-coated peppermint oil in the irritable bowel syndrome: A randomized double-blind crossover study. *J Gastroenterol Hepatol* 3: 235–238, 1988.

8. Carling L, et al. Short-term treatment of the irritable bowel syndrome: A placebo controlled trial of peppermint oil against hyoscyaminme. *Opuscula Medica* 34: 55–57, 1989.

9. Spindler P, et al. Subchronic toxicity study of peppermint oil in rats. *Toxicol Lett* 62: 215–220, 1992.

10. ESCOP monographs. Fascicule 3: *Menthae Piperitae Aetheroleum* (peppermint oil). Exeter, UK: ESCOP, 1997: 1–6.

11. ESCOP. 1997: 5.

Pygeum

1. Schulz V, et al. Rational phytotherapy. New York: Springer-Verlag, 1998: 232.

2. Schulz V, et al. 1998: 233.

3. Duvia R, et al. Advances in the phytotherapy of prostatic hypertrophy. *Med Pr* 4: 143–148, 1983.

4. Schulz V, et al. 1998: 233.

Red Clover

1. Newall C, et al. Herbal medicines: A guide for health-care professionals. London: Pharmaceutical Press, 1996: 227.

2. Yanagihara K, et al. Antiproliferative effects of isoflavones on human cancer cell lines established from the gastrointestinal tract. *Cancer Res* 53: 5815–5821, 1993.

Red Raspberry

1. Bamford DS, et al. Raspberry leaf tea: A new aspect to an old problem. *Br J Pharmacol* 40: 161–162, 1970.

Saw Palmetto

1. Nickel JC. Placebo therapy of benign prostatic hyperplasia: A 25-month study. *Br J Urol* 81: 383–387, 1988.

2. Braeckman J. The extract of *Serenoa repens* in the treatment of benign prostatic hyperplasia: A multicenter open study. *Curr Ther Res* 55: 776–785, 1994.

3. Romics I, Schmitz H, and Frang D. Experience in treating benign prostatic hypertrophy with *Sabal serrulata* for one year. *Int Urol Nephrol* 25: 565–569, 1993.

4. Emili E, et al. Clinical trial of a new drug for treating hypertrophy of the prostate (Permixon). *Urologia* 50: 1042–1048, 1983.

5. Champault G, et al. A double-blind trial of an extract of the plant *Serenoa repens* in benign prostatic hyperplasia. *Br J Clin Pharmacol* 18(3): 461–462, 1984.

6. Tasca A, et al. Treatment of obstructive symptomatology caused by prostatic adenoma with an extract of *Serenoa repens*. Double-blind clinical study vs. placebo. *Minerva Urol Nefrol* 37(1): 87–91, 1985.

7. Boccafoschi S et al. Comparison of *Serenoa repens* extract with placebo by controlled clinical trial in patients with prostatic adenomatosis. *Urologia* 50: 1257–1268, 1983.

8. Smith RH, et al. The value of Permixon in benign prostatic hypertrophy. *Br J Urol* 58:36–40, 1986.

9. Descotes JL, et al. Placebo-controlled evaluation of the efficacy and tolerability of Permixon in benign prostatic hyperplasia after exclusion of placebo responders. *Clin Drug Invest* 9: 291–297, 1995.

10. Mattei FM, et al. *Serenoa repens* extract in the medical treatment of benign prostatic hypertrophy. *Urologia* 55: 547–552, 1988.

11. Plosker GL, et al. *Serenoa repens* (Permixon). A review of its pharmacology and therapeutic efficacy in benign prostatic hyperplasia. *Drugs Aging* 9(5): 379–395, 1996.

12. Carraro J, et al. Comparison of phytotherapy (Permixon) with finasteride in the treatment of benign prostate hyperplasia: A randomized international study of 1,098 patients. *Prostate* 29(4): 231–240, 241–242, 1996.

13. Bach D. Medikamentosse Langzeitbehandlung der BPH. Ergebnisse einer prospektiven 3-Jahresstudie mit dem Sabal extrakt IDS 89. *Urologe B* 35: 178–183, 1995.

14. Bach D, et al. Phytopharmaceutical and synthetic agents in the treatment of benign prostatic hyperplasia (BPH). *Phytomedicine* 3(4): 309–313, 1997.

15. Braeckman J, et al. Efficacy and safety of the extract of *Serenoa repens* in the treatment of benign prostatic hyperplasia: The therapeutic equivalence between twice and once daily dosage forms. *Phytother Res* 11(8): 558–563, 1997.

16. Plosker GL, et al. 1996.

17. Plosker GL, et al. 1996.

18. Bach D, et al. 1997.

Sitosterol

1. Schulz V, et al. Rational phytotherapy. New York: Springer-Verlag, 1998: 231.

2. Pegel K. The importance of sitosterol and sitosterolin in human and animal nutrition. *S African J Science* 93: 263–268, 1997.

3. Berges B, et al. Randomised, placebo-controlled, double-blind clinical trial of beta-sitosterol in patients with benign prostatic hyperplasia. *Lancet* 345: 1529–1532, 1995.

4. Schulz V, et al. 1998.

5. Berges B, et al. 1995.

Skullcap

1. Newall C, et al. Herbal medicines: A guide for health-care professionals. London: Pharmaceutical Press, 1996: 239.

Slippery Elm

1. Castleman M. The healing herbs. Emmaus, PA: Rodale Press, 1991: 342–344.

Stevia

1. Leung A, et al. Encyclopedia of common natural ingredients used in foods, drugs, and costmetics. New York: John Wiley and Sons, 1996.

2. Kinghorn D, et al. Current status of stevioside as a sweetening agent for human use. Economics and Medicinal Plant Research. Vol. I. London: Academic Press, Inc. Ltd, 1985.

3. Leung A, et al. 1996.

St. John's Wort

1. Suzuki O, et al. Inhibition of monoamine oxidase by hypericin. *Planta Med* 50: 2722–2724, 1984.

2. Bladt S, et al. Inhibition of MAO by fractions and constituents of hypericum extract. *J Geriatr Psychiatry Neurol* 7(Suppl. 1): S57–S59, 1994.

3. Thiede B, et al. Inhibition of MAO and COMT by hypericum extracts and hypericin. *J Geriatr Psychiatry Neurol* 7(Suppl. 1): 54–56, 1994.

4. Muller WEG, et al. Effects of hypericum extract on the expression of serotonin receptors. *J Geriatr Psychiatry Neurol* 7(Suppl. 1): S63–S64, 1994.

5. Muller WE, et al. Hypericum extract (LI160) as an herbal antidepressant. *Pharmacopsychiatry* 30(Suppl. 2): 71–134, 1997.

6. Hansgen KD, et al. Multicenter double-blind study examining the antidepressant effectiveness of the hypericum extract LI 160. *J Geriatr Psychiatry Neurol* 7(Suppl. 1): S15–S18, 1994.

7. Laakman G, et al. St. John's wort in mild to moderate depression: The relevance of hyperforin for the clinical efficacy. *Pharmacopsychiatry* 31(Suppl.): 54–59, 1998.

8. Linde K, et al. St. John's wort for depression—An overview and meta-analysis of randomized clinical trials. *Br Med J* 313: 253–258, 1996.

9. Ernst E. St. John's wort, an anti-depressant? A systematic, criteria-based review. *Phytomedicine* 2(1): 67–71, 1995.

10. Schulz V, et al. Rational phytotherapy. New York: Springer-Verlag, 1998: 59.

11. Linde K, et al. 1996.

12. Ernst E. 1995.

13. Vorbach EU, et al. Efficacy and tolerability of St. John's wort extract LI 160 vs. imipramine in patients with severe depressive episodes according to ICD-10. *Pharmacopsychiatry* 30(Suppl. 2): 81–85, 1997.

14. Martinez B, et al. Hypericum in the treatment of seasonal affective disorders. *J Geriatr Psychiatry Neurol* 7(Suppl. 1): 29–33, 1994.

15. Woelk H, et al. Benefits and risks of the hypericum extract LI 160: Drug monitoring study with 3,250 patients. *J Geriatr Psychiatry Neurol* 7(Suppl 1): S34–S38, 1994.

16. Smet P and Nolen W. St. John's wort as an anti-depressant. *Br Med J* 3: 241–242, 1996.

17. Schulz V, et al. 1998: 56.

18. Seigers CP, et al. Phototoxicity caused by hypericum. *Nervenhielkunde* 12: 320–322, 1993.

19. Brockmoller J, et al. Hypericin and pseudohypericin: Pharmacokinetics and effects on photosensitivity in humans. *Pharmacopsychiatry* 30(Suppl. 2): 94–101, 1997.

20. Suzuki O, et al. 1984.

21. Bladt S, et al. 1994.

22. Thiede B, et al. 1994.

23. Nebel A, Baker RK, and Kroll DJ. Potential metabolic interaction between theophylline and St. John's wort. Submitted to *Annals of Pharmacotherapy,* 1998.

24. Baker RK, Sampey B, and Kroll DJ. Catalytic inhibition of human DNA topoisomerase II alpha by hypericin, a naphthodianthone from St. John's wort *(Hypericum perforatum).* Manuscript in preparation.

Suma

1. De Oliveira F. *Pfaffia paniculata* (Martius) Kuntze- Brazilian ginseng. *Rev Bras Farmacog* 1(1): 86–92, 1986.

Tea Tree

1. Williams LR, et al. The composition and bactericidal activity of oil of *Melaleuca alternifolia* (tea tree oil). *Int J Aromather* 1(3): 15, 1989.

2. Bassett IB, et al. *Med J Aust* 153: 455–458, 1990.

Turmeric

1. Ammon HPT, et al. Pharmacology of *Curcuma longa*. *Planta Med* 57: 1–7, 1991.

2. Sreejayan N, et al. Free radical scavenging activity of curcuminoids. *Arzneimittelforschung Drug Res* 46: 169–171, 1996.

3. Deodhar SD, et al. Preliminary studies on antirheumatic activity of curcumin. *Indian J Med Res* 71: 632–634, 1980.

4. Ravindranath V, et al. Absorption and tissue distribution of curcumin in rats. *Toxicology* 16: 259–265, 1980.

5. Ammon HPT, et al. 1991.

6. Shankar TNB, et al. Toxicity studies on turmeric (*Cucurma longa*): Acute toxicity studies in rats, guinea pigs and monkeys. *Indian J Exp Biol* 18: 73–75, 1980.

Uva Ursi

1. Frohne V, et al. Untersuchungen zur Frage der harndesifizierenden Wirkungen von Barentraubenblatt-extracten. *Planta Med* 18: 1–25, 1970.

2. Tyler V. Herbs of choice. New York: Pharmaceutical Products Press, 1994: 79.

3. Leung A, et al. Encyclopedia of common natural ingredients used in food, drugs, and cosmetics, 2nd ed. New York: John Wiley and Sons, 1996: 505.

4. ESCOP monographs. Fascicule 5: *Uvae Ursi Folium*. Exeter, UK: ESCOP, 1997.

5. Schulz V, et al. Rational phytotherapy. New York: Springer-Verlag, 1998: 223.

6. Frohne V, et al. 1970.

7. Kedzia B, et al. Antibacterial action of urine containing arbutin metabolic products. *Med Dosw Mikrobiol* 27: 305–314, 1975.

8. Larsson B, et al. Prophylactic effect of UVA-E in women with recurrent cystitis: A preliminary report. *Curr Ther Res* 53: 441–443, 1993.

9. ESCOP. 1997.

10. Tyler V. Herbs of choice. New York: Pharmaceutical Products Press, 1994: 79.

11. Schulz V, et al. Rational phytotherapy. New York: Springer-Verlag, 1998: 224.

12. Nowak AK, et al. Darkroom hepatitis after exposure to hydroquinone. *Lancet* 345: 1187, 1995.

13. U.S. Environmental Protection Agency. Extremely hazardous substances. Superfund chemical profiles. Park Ridge NJ: Noyes Data Corporation, 1988: 1906–1907.

14. Lewis RJ. Sax's dangerous properties of industrial materials, 8th ed. New York: Van Nostrand Reinhold, 1989: 1906–1907.

15. Schulz V, et al. 1998: 223.

Valerian

1. Houghton PF. The biological activity of valerian and related plants. *J Ethnopharmacol* 22(2): 121–142, 1988.

2. Krieglstein J, et al. Valepotriate, valenrensaure, valeranon und atherisches 01 sind jedoch unwirksam. Zentraldampfende inhaltsstoffe im baldrian. *Deutsch Apoth Z* 128: 2041–2046, 1988.

3. Holzl J, et al. Receptor binding studies with *Valeriana officinalis* on the benzodiazepine receptor. *Planta Med* 55: 642, 1989.

4. Mennini T, et al. In vitro study on the interaction of extracts and pure compounds from *Valeriana officinalis* roots with

GABA, benzodiazepine, and barbiturate receptors in rat brain. *Fitoterapia* 54: 291–300, 1993.

5. Schulz V, et al. Rational phytotherapy. New York: Springer-Verlag, 1998: 75–76.

6. Cavadas C, et al. In vitro study on the interaction of *Valeriana officinalis* L. Extracts and their amino acids on GABA(A) receptor in rat brain. *Arzneimittelforschung* 45(7): 753–755, 1995.

7. Schulz V, et al. 1998: 81.

8. Schulz V, et al. 1998: 78–80.

9. Lindahl O, et al. Double blind study of a valerian preparation. *Pharmacol Biochem Behav* 32(4): 1065–1066, 1989.

10. ESCOP monographs. Fascicule 4: *Valerianae radix*. Exeter, UK: ESCOP, 1997: 5–6.

11. Leathwood PD, et al. Aqueous extract of valerian root (*Valeriana officinalis* L.) improves sleep quality in man. *Pharmacol Biochem Behav* 17(1): 65–71, 1982.

12. Dressing H, et al. Insomnia: Are valerian/balm combinations of equal value to benzodiazepine? *Therapiewoche* 42: 726–736, 1992.

13. Kohnen R, et al. The effects of valerian, propranolol, and their combination on activation, performance and mood of healthy volunteers under social stress conditions. *Pharmacopsychiatry* 21: 447–448, 1988.

14. Hendriks H, et al. Central nervous depressant activity of valerenic acid in the mouse. *Planta Med* 51: 28–31, 1985.

15. Leuschner J, et al. Characterization of the central nervous depressant activity of a commercially available valerian root extract. *Arzneimittelforschung* 43(6): 638–641, 1993.

16. Krieglstein J, et al. Valepotriate, valenrensaure, valeranon und atherisches 01 sind jedoch unwirksam. Zentraldampfende inhaltsstoffe im baldrian. *Deutsch Apoth Z* 128: 2041–2046, 1988.

17. ESCOP. 1997: 3–4.

18. Schulz V, et al. 1998: 77, 81.

19. Rosecrans JA, et al. Pharmacological investigation of certain *Valeriana officinalis* L. extracts. *J Pharmacol Sci* 50: 240–244, 1996.

20. Tyler V. Herbs of choice. New York: Pharmaceutical Products Press, 1994: 118.

21. ESCOP. 1997: 1.

22. Schulz V, et al. 1998: 77, 81.

23. Albrecht M, et al. Psychopharmaceuticals and safety in traffic. *Z Allg Med* 71: 1215–1221, 1995.

24. Gerhard U, et al. Vigilance-decreasing effects of two plant-derived sedatives. *Schweiz Rundsch Med Prax* 85(15): 473–481, 1996.

25. ESCOP. 1997: 2.

26. ESCOP. 1997: 2.

27. Albrecht M, et al. 1995.

28. Sakamoto T, et al. Psychotropic effects of Japanese valerian root extract. *Chem Pharm Bull (Tokyo)* 40(3): 758–761, 1992.

White Willow

1. Newall C, et al. Herbal medicines: A guide for health-care professionals. London: Pharmaceutical Press, 1996: 268.

2. Lininger S, et al. The natural pharmacy. Rocklin, CA: Prima Publishing, 1998: 319.

Wild Yam

1. Lininger S, et al. The natural pharmacy. Rocklin, CA: Prima Publishing, 1998: 320.

2. Tierra M. The way of herbs. New York: Pocket Books, 1990: 246.

3. Tyler V, et al. Pharmacognosy, 8th ed. Philadelphia, PA: Lea & Febiger, 1981.

4. Hudson TND. Townsend letter for doctors and patients. Port Townsend, WA, 1996, Issue No. 156.

Yarrow

1. Newall C, et al. Herbal medicines: A guide for health-care professionals. London: Pharmaceutical Press, 1996: 272.

Yerba Santa

1. Lawrence Review of Natural Products. Yerba santa monograph. St. Louis, MO: Facts and Comparisons, Division, J.B. Lipincott Company, 1991.

2. Tierra M. The way of herbs. New York: Pocket Books, 1990: 254.

3. Lawrence Review of Natural Products. 1991.

Yohimbe

1. Riley AJ. Yohimbine in the treatment of erectile disorder. *Br J Clin Pract* 48(3): 133–136, 1994.

2. Riley AJ. 1994.

3. Lawrence Review of Natural Products. Yohimbe monograph. St. Louis, MO: Facts and Comparisons Division, J.B. Lipincott Company,1993.

Yucca

1. Bingham R, et al. Yucca plant saponin in the management of arthritis. *J Appl Nutr* 27(2–3): 45–51, 1975.

Chinese Herbal Combinations

Bi Yan Pian/Pe Min Kan Wan

1. Zhu Chun-Han. Clinical handbook of Chinese prepared medicines. Brookline, MA: Paradigm Publications, 1989: 53.

2. M&A Natural Healthcare Products Co., Ltd. Product Insert. Shatin, Hong Kong.

3. Zhu Chun-Han. 1989.

Curing Pills/Po Chai

1. Zhu Chun-Han. Clinical handbook of Chinese prepared medicines. Brookline, MA: Paradigm Publications, 1989: 63.

Yin Ciao

1. Zhu Chun-Han. Clinical handbook of Chinese prepared medicines. Brookline, MA: Paradigm Publications, 1989: 46–47.

Index

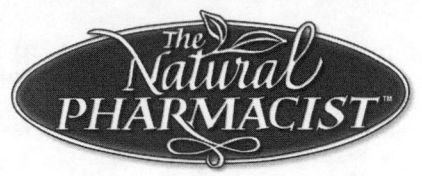

About the Series Editors

Steven Bratman, M.D., medical director of Prima Health, has many years of experience in the alternative medicine field. A graduate of the University of California at Davis, Medical School, he has also trained in herbology, nutrition, Chinese medicine, and other alternative therapies, and has worked closely with a wide variety of alternative practitioners. He is the author of *The Natural Pharmacist: Your Complete Guide to Illnesses and Their Natural Remedies* (Prima), *The Natural Pharmacist Guide to St. John's Wort and Depression* (Prima), *The Alternative Medicine Ratings Guide* (Prima), and *The Alternative Medicine Sourcebook* (Lowell House).

David J. Kroll, Ph.D., is a professor of pharmacology and toxicology at the University of Colorado School of Pharmacy and a consultant for pharmacists, physicians, and alternative practitioners on the indications and cautions for herbal medicine use. A graduate of both the University of Florida and the Philadelphia College of Pharmacy and Science, Dr. Kroll has lectured widely and has published article in a number of medical journals, abstracts, and newsletters.